How to Read Lips
for Fun and Profit

EDWARD B. NITCHIE

How to Read Lips for Fun and Profit

Illustrations by Mike McIver

HAWTHORN BOOKS, INC.
Publishers / New York
A Howard & Wyndham Company

HOW TO READ LIPS FOR FUN AND PROFIT

Library of Congress Catalog Card Number: 78-65386
ISBN: 0-8015-3740-1
1 2 3 4 5 6 7 8 9 10

How to Read Lips
for Fun and Profit

Study and Practice

ONE WORD OF WARNING—this book is not an end, but a means to an end. That end is that those who study the book may, by watching others' lips, be able to understand what is said. So the student must not look upon the lessons, explanations, and remarks as things to be memorized, but only as things to make the subject in hand clear and so help the ultimate end. So, too, the systems of symbols used in the book are a means to the ultimate end and not an end in themselves. Therefore I would say to the student, do not let the apparent amount and difficulty of the work (due to present unfamiliarity with it) discourage you or turn you aside from the study. Take only a little at a time, and results are certain. Do not forget, too, that results will not come overnight; there will be no miracle. If you were taking music lessons, you would expect to practice faithfully and wait the combined result of time and practice to bring perfection. So must it be with any study, and lipreading is no exception.

Your study and practice should be of two kinds; practice by yourself with the mirror, and practice with your friends. Each type of practice has its own peculiar value and cannot be fully substituted by the other. Mirror practice is most valuable at the outset of the study, but practice with friends assumes an increasingly dominant importance as the work proceeds.

MIRROR PRACTICE

There are eighteen positions assumed by the *visible* organs of speech in making the different sounds found in the English language. The aim and value of mirror practice is so to fix these eighteen positions in mind that the recognition of them and the association of them with the sounds they severally cover shall become automatic and spontaneous. To accomplish this, study as follows:

Each position is carefully described. With this description are printed two illustrations of the position, one being for a woman's face and one for a man's. Read the description and observe the position as shown in the drawings. Then form the sounds covered by the position with your own lips and observe the position in the mirror.

Then read the remarks. They are given you merely as a help to making everything clear.

After the remarks, a summary of the position is given to help you fix the *essential* points in your mind.

With the positions, words and sentences are given that contain only positions already studied. This is important inasmuch as associated positions have a greater or less modifying effect on positions connected with them.

Take the words given and pronounce them to yourself before the mirror. Study *down* the column, not across the page. As you pronounce the words, observe carefully the position assumed for each sound in the words. I realize that it is more or less difficult to do this, for the pupil, knowing what is said, is tempted to let the mind wander, and thus the value of mirror practice is lost. To overcome this difficulty I have devised a system of symbols to represent each position. Each position has a *name* descriptive of its cardinal point of individuality. The symbol used is an *abbreviation* of this name. Therefore the symbol has a *significance*, and if the pupil as he studies the words before the mirror writes down the symbol for each position as he comes to it, he compels himself not only to keep his attention fixed, but also to think of this cardinal point individualizing the position observed. Because the symbols have a significance and a meaning, they will be found easy to remember.

The pupil, then, should pronounce each word naturally before the mirror, observing the position for each sound in the word, and writing down the symbol for the position at the same time. When writing the symbols, think always of the *name* of the position of which the symbol is the abbreviation. The pupil must remember in this part of the work *always to use the mirror.*

In studying sentences, pursue much the same method as directed for studying the words, except *do not* pronounce the sentences word by word: for example, "I-lost-a-dollar-from-my-purse," for if you do you will make the pronunciations of some of the words very artificial. It is necessary that the words should be pronounced naturally as in ordinary conversation. Therefore, pronounce the words in their natural groups, "I lost a dollar—from my purse," studying and writing down the symbols for one group at a time.

Following the sentences, a study is given in turning words and sentences (represented by their symbols) back into English. This work should be done also with the mirror; the pupils forming the positions as indicated by the symbols and then from their own lips deciphering the words and sentences.

PRACTICE WITH FRIENDS

After you have finished the mirror practice in a lesson, ask a friend to read to you the words and sentences given in that lesson. The voice of your friend must be absolutely inaudible to you, so that you are entirely dependent upon your eyes for understanding what is said. All practice with friends must be of this inaudible kind.

SOME GENERAL SUGGESTIONS

At the beginning of each of the first fifteen lessons a brief review is given of the two preceding lessons. This is merely to help the pupil keep the cardinal points in mind.

The pupil must observe particularly that "sounds and letters disagree," and that it is the sounds and not the letters that are basic, and that form the positions. Further explanations are given with each position.

The eighteen positions are learned in fifteen lessons. Twenty lessons follow these, giving special drill exercises, and further applications of the positions, as is fully explained with the positions.

SOME DON'TS

Don't forget to use the mirror.
Don't do your work carelessly.
Don't try to do too much at a time.
Don't study more than one hour at a sitting.
Don't expect results unless you work for them.
Don't forget to make your pronunciations as natural as possible.
Don't in any case be discouraged, but keep everlastingly at it
      until you win.

SOME DOS

Do study faithfully.
Do study regularly.
Do study at least one hour a day.
Do keep at it until you succeed.

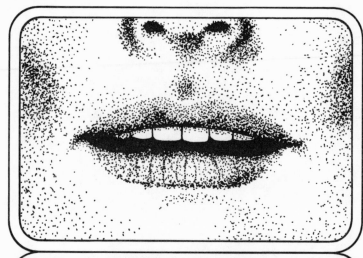

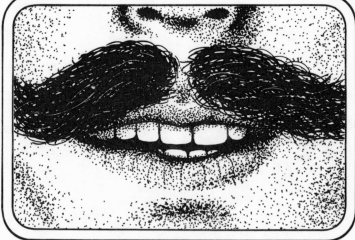

Position First

Position First (na)

For the sound of long $\bar{e}$ (as in "we") the lips assume a *narrow*, slitlike opening, and the corners of the mouth are slightly drawn back and parted.

REMARKS

1. Observe that it is not necessary to have the letter *e* to have the long $\bar{e}$ sound. For example, the *ie* in "brief," the *i* in "ceiling," the *ea* in "cease," the *ee* in "free"—all have the sound of long $\bar{e}$. Thus the vowels in each of the words given show Position First regardless of the letters.

2. This position is called the "narrow" position, and is represented by the abbreviation *na* (for "*na*rrow").

3. The sound of the aspirate *h* shows no facial position whatever, and the effect of the sound in ordinary speech is not appreciable in outward appearance.* Therefore the word "he" resolves itself into one facial element represented by the abbreviation *na*. That is, when the word "he" is pronounced, the lips assume the narrow, slitlike opening described above.

Summary of Position First:
>   *The sound is a long $\bar{e}$.*
>   *The facial appearance is a "narrow" mouth.*
>   *The symbol of representation is na.*

---

*H is, moreover, the only sound which has no appreciable outward effect.

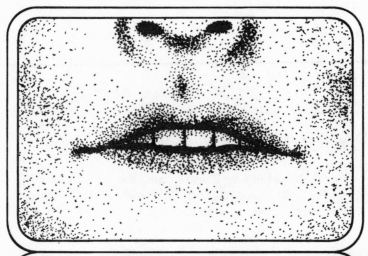

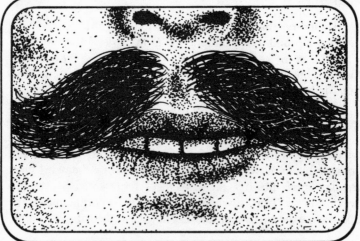

Position Second

Position Second (lt)

For the sounds represented by the letters *f* (as in "few") and *v* (as in "view") the lower *lip* rises and touches the upper *teeth*.*

REMARKS

1. Observe that *ph* in "sylph" has the sound of *f*, and that *ph* in "Stephen" has the sound of *v*. Thus *ph* in these and similar words will show Position Second. So, too, *gh* in "rough," etc., has the sound of *f*, and shows Position Second.

2. This position is called the "lip-to-teeth" position, and is represented by the abbreviation *lt* (for "*lip-to-teeth*").

Summary of Position Second:
  The sounds are represented by f and v.
  The facial appearance is "lip-to-teeth."
  The symbol of representation is lt.

We are now in a position to take certain words of two sounds and resolve them into their component facial elements, using the mirror, and then representing on paper each element seen in the mirror by its appropriate abbreviation, as follows:

fee = *lt-na*   eve = *na-lt*   heave = *na-lt*

Position Third (ls)

For the sounds represented by the letters *p* (as in "pea"), *b* (as in "bee"), and *m* (as in "me"), the *lips* are *shut* naturally, as when the face is in repose.

---

*Many of the positions cover more than one sound. Though this is confusing for single words, the words when put in a sentence will usually be revealed by the sense of the sentence.

REMARKS

1. At the end of a word spoken alone, *p* and *b* will show a slight difference from *m*, in that the mouth opens for *p* and *b*, and remains closed for *m*. But at the beginning of a word, or in middle of a word, or at the end of a word which stands in the middle of a sentence, the mouth naturally opens immediately after an *m* sound for forming the following sound, so that, except at the end of a sentence, *p*, *b*, and *m* will all show precisely the same position.

2. This position is called the "lip-shut" position, and is represented by the abbreviation *ls* (for "*l*ip-shut").

Summary of Position Third:
> *The sounds are represented by p, b, and m.*
> *The facial appearance is "lip-shut."*
> *The symbol of representation is ls.*

Resolve the following words into their component facial elements:

pea = *ls-na*	beef	peep
bee	heap	beam

Resolve the following positions into words:

na-lt = eve	*ls-na* = pea
lt-na	*ls-na-lt*

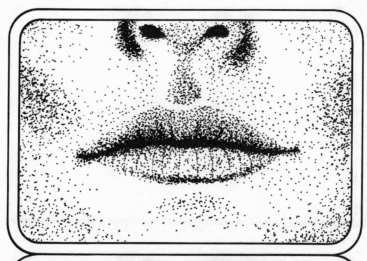

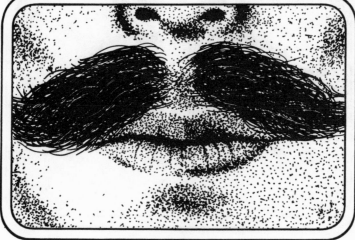

Position Third

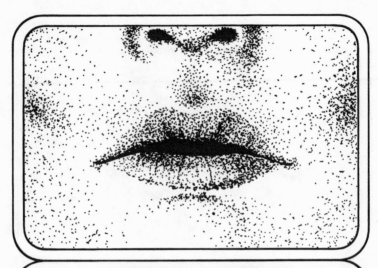

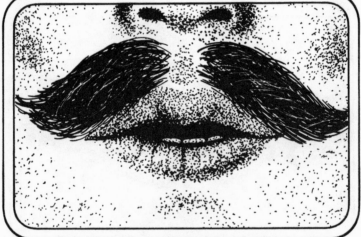

Position Fourth

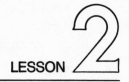

Review of Preceding Lesson:

Position	Sounds	Facial Appearance	Symbol
1st	long ē	"narrow" mouth	*na*
2nd	f, v	"lip-to-teeth"	*lt*
3rd	p, b, m	"lip-shut"	*ls*

Position Fourth *(pu)*

For the sound of long $\overline{oo}$ (as in "moon") the lips are *puckered*, showing the smallest opening of the mouth of any of the positions. The lips, however, are not puckered as much as in whistling.

REMARKS

1. Observe that the long $\overline{oo}$ sound occurs for the *o* in "prove," for the *ou* in "youth," for the *u* in "rude," etc., and that all these vowels therefore show Position Fourth.

2. This position is called the "puckered" position, and is represented by the abbreviation *pu* (for "*puckered*").

Summary of Position Fourth:
> *The sound is long $\overline{oo}$.*
> *The facial appearance is a "puckered" mouth.*
> *The symbol of representation is pu.*

Resolve the following words:

    boo = *ls-pu*   poop   who = *pu**
    move   boom

Resolve into words:

    ls-pu-lt   *ls-pu-ls*

General Remark

Throughout the previous positions we have considered the vowel sounds as accented, or stressed, vowel sounds. In certain of the positions to follow we shall speak especially of unaccented, or unstressed, vowel sounds. In the English language a change of accent or stress often makes a marked change in sound, and this marked change in sound usually makes a vital change in the visible facial position. This is a matter which has hitherto never been adequately presented in any method or system of lipreading. If lipreading is to have value it must pay special attention to the positions of ordinary colloquial speech (not stilted or "vocabulary" speech), and it must study in particular the positions as affected in ordinary speech by lack of accent or stress.

Position Fifth *(so)*

For the sound of short $\breve{o}\breve{o}$ (as in "good") and for the sounds represented by the letters *w* (as in "we"), and *wh* (as in "wharf") the lips assume the position of a *small oval*. The lips are noticeably less puckered than for the preceding position for long $\overline{oo}$.

---

*Observe that in this word *wh* has the sound of *h*, and "who" is sounded "hoo," thus showing merely the "puckered" position.

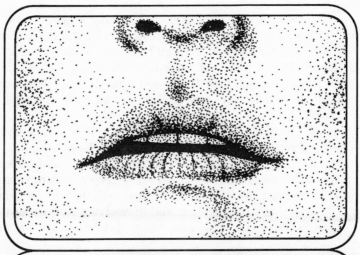

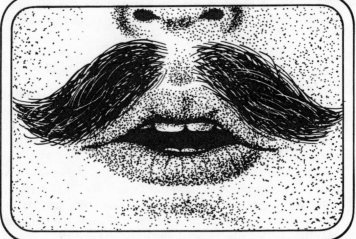

Position Fifth

REMARKS

1. Observe that the sound of the *u* after *q* (as in "queen," which equals "kween"), is the sound of a *w*, and hence shows Position Fifth. Also, observe that the short ŏŏ sound occurs frequently for *u* (as in "put"), for *ou* (as in "should"), and for *o* (as in "wolf"), and that these vowels, therefore, show the same position as short ŏŏ. Observe, further that *oo* before *r* (as in "poor") has the short ŏŏ sound.

2. This position is called the "small-oval" position, and is represented by the abbreviation *so* (for "small-*o*val").

3. There are a number of words, such as "hoof, "roof," "hoop," "room," etc., which by some people are pronounced with the short ŏŏ sound, and by others with the long ŏŏ sound. In mirror practice, therefore, and in resolving such words into their symbols, students must be guided by their own pronunciation.

4. It will be of service to contrast the "small-oval" of short ŏŏ with the "puckered" mouth of long ŏŏ, as follows:

foot	put	full	pull
food	boot	fool	pool

5. Unaccented *u* in a final -ful, -ure, etc. (as "beautiful," "future") will, in careful pronunciation, show this "small-oval"; but more colloquially this *u* sound will be like unaccented short ŭ and hence will show the "elliptical" mouth to be described later under Position Seventh.)

6. The *o* in the preposition "to" and in the auxiliary verb "do," *in a sentence*, will show this "small-oval" (*so*) position; or if the words are carelessly spoken (as is not infrequent) with the sound of unaccented short ŭ, the *o* will show the "elliptical" mouth to be described later under Position Seventh.

Summary of Position Fifth:
>   *The sounds are represented by short ŏŏ, w, wh.*
>   *The facial appearance is a "small-oval."*
>   *The symbol of representation is so.*

Resolve:

we = *so-na*	weep	hoof
weave	woo	hoop

We weave = *so-na so-na-lt.*

We woo.	We weep.
We whoop.	We move.

Resolve:

so-na-ls = weep	*so-na-lt*
so-pu	*so-na*

Position Sixth *(wi)*

For the sound of Italian *a* (as in "farm") the mouth is opened *widely*, more widely than for any other sound. The mouth, however, is not opened as widely as in yawning. The tongue is slightly drawn back in the mouth.

REMARKS

1. This Italian sound of *a* occurs before silent *l* (as in "palm") and commonly before *r* (as in "farm"), and in a few other words, such as "father."

2. This position is called the "wide" position, and is represented by the abbreviation *wi* (for "*wi*de").

3. The *a* in such words as "pass," "last," "ask," etc., is not infrequently heard with this Italian *a* sound, and when so pronounced will show Position Sixth, the "wide" (*wi* position. Otherwise it will show a position to be described later.*

4. The sound of short *ŏ* (as in "odd") is quite frequently

---

*When letters in the same words are sounded differently by different people, they will not enter into the practice words and sentences until all the positions which they may show have been studied.

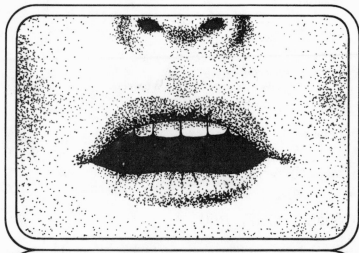

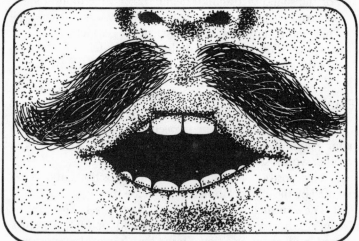

Position Sixth

heard, as an extreme short sound of Italian *a*, and when so pronounced will show Position Sixth. Short ŏ is also commonly heard as an extreme short sound of broad *a* (*aw*), and when so pronounced shows the same position as broad *a* to be described later.

Summary of Position Sixth:
> *The sound is Italian a (ah).*
> *The facial appearance is a "wide" mouth.*
> *The symbol of representation is wi.*

Resolve:

> alm = *wi-ls*   palm   balm

Resolve:

> *ls-wi-ls*

Review of Preceding Lessons 1 and 2

Position	Sounds	Facial Appearance	Symbol
1st	long ē	"narrow" mouth	*na*
2nd	f, v	"lip-to-teeth"	*lt*
3rd	p, b, m	"lip-shut"	*ls*
4th	long ō͞o	"puckered" mouth	*pu*
5th	short ŏ͝o, w, wh	"small-oval"	*so*
6th	Italian a (ah)	"wide" mouth	*wi*

The diphthongal sound of *ow* (as in "cow") shows a combination of Positions Sixth and Fifth, that is, of the "wide" (*wi*) and the "small-oval" (*so*) positions, the former shading into the latter.

REMARKS

1. The letters *ou* (as in "out") frequently have the same sound as *ow*, and hence will show the same combination of positions.

2. This combination of positions is represented by a combination of the symbols, thus, *wi-so*.

Resolve:

vow = *lt-wi-so*   wow
bough   bow-wow
We vow. = *so-na lt-wi-so.*
We bow.

Resolve:

ls-wi-so   so-wi-so

General Summary of Position Sixth:
Italian a (ah) = "*wide*" *mouth* = *wi.*
ow = "*wide*" *plus* "*small-oval*" = *wi-so.*

Position Seventh *(el)*

For the sound of accented short *ŭ* (as in "up"), unaccented short *ŭ* (as in "upon"), and *u* before *r*, (as in
"fur"), the mouth is neither narrowly nor widely
opened, but assumes an intermediate position with an
elliptical shape.

REMARKS

1. Observe that the sound of accented short *ŭ* occurs sometimes for letters other than *u*. For example, the *ou* in "enough,"
and the *o* in "love" have the sound of short *u*, and hence show
this Position Seventh.
2. Observe that the sound of unaccented short *ŭ* occurs
commonly in ordinary speech for other unaccented letters. For
example, the unaccented *a* in "around," the final *a* in "Russia,"
the unaccented *a* in the terminations -al (loyal), -able (capable),
-ance (balance), etc., the vowel in final unaccented -er (farmer),
-or (parlor), -yr (martyr), etc., and the unaccented *o* in "occasion," "compel," etc., all colloquially have the sound of unaccented short *ŭ*, and hence show this Position Seventh.
3. The sound of *u* before *r* as in "fur" occurs also for the *i* in
"fir" and the *e* in "her," etc., and hence these vowels also
show this Position Seventh.
4. This position is called the "elliptical" position, and is
represented by the abbreviation *el* (for "*el*liptical").
5. A number of the auxiliary words in the English language
are, when occurring in a sentence, practically equivalent to unaccented syllables, being unstressed, and more or less slurred.

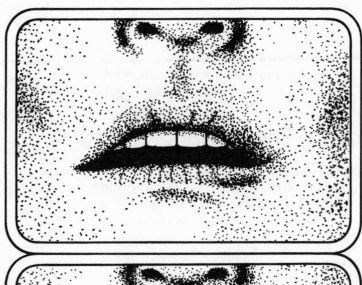

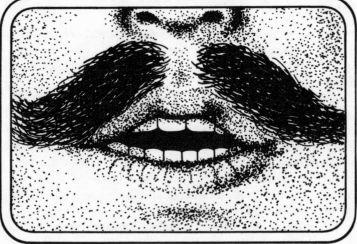

Position Seventh

So the articles "a" and "an," and the conjunction "and," *when occurring in a sentence*, usually have the vowel sound of unaccented short ŭ, showing the "elliptical" position. The same sound and position also occur in the definite article "the" when the next word begins with a consonant sound.

And again, the vowel sound in the auxiliary verbs, such as "has" and "had," is colloquially heard in a sentence as an unaccented short *u* sound, showing the "elliptical" position. This will be made clear by contrasting the difference in sound in the two "hads" of the sentence, "I had had it," which sounds like "I hud had it."

6. See also remarks 5 and 6 under Position Fifth.

Summary of Position Seventh:
> *The sounds are short ŭ, and u in "fur."*
> *The facial appearance is an "elliptical" mouth.*
> *The symbol of representation is el.*

Resolve:

huff = *el-lt*	hub	pup
muff	hum	pump
puff	hump = *el-* + *ls**	bump

We puff. = *so-na ls-el-lt*
We pump.
Bump me.

Resolve:

ls-el-ls = mum	*ls-el-* + *ls*	*el-ls*
ls-el-lt	*el-lt*	*el-* + *ls*

---

*What may be called a "time-element" enters into the visible facial positions quite frequently. It occurs where there are two distinct and different sounds coming together, each of which happens to require the same position. Thus in the word "hump" we have an *m* and a *p* sound coming together and each of these sounds require the "lip-shut" position. As these two sounds are not, and cannot be, sounded simultaneously, the result is that the "lip-shut" position is held for a longer time for the two sounds than it would be held for either one of the sounds alone. This "time-element" is represented by prefixing a plus sign (+) to the symbol of abbreviation. Thus, "hump" = *el-* + *ls*. Contrast with this, "hub" = *el-ls*.

Review of Preceding Lessons 2 and 3

Position	Sounds	Facial Appearance	Symbol
4th	long o͞o	"puckered" mouth	*pu*
5th	short o̯o̯, w, wh	"small-oval"	*so*
6th	Italian a (ah)	"wide" mouth	*wi*
6th-5th	ow	"wide" plus "small-oval"	*wi-so*
7th	short ŭ, u in "fur"	"elliptical" mouth	*el*

Position Eighth *(ep)*

For the sound represented by the letter *r* (as in "free"), there is an *elliptical* position of the lips somewhat as for Position Seventh, with the important difference that for *r* the corners of the mouth are slightly *puckered*.

REMARKS

1. Further aids to the quick recognition of this position are (a) that the lower lip and chin are slightly forward (this is what gives the "pucker" to the corners of the mouth), and (b) that if the tongue is visible (as it will be under a good light), the point of the tongue will be seen to curve upwards in the mouth.

2. This position is called the "elliptical-puckered" position, and is represented by the abbreviation *ep* (for "elliptical-puckered").

3. *R* is the most variable sound in the English language in the strength with which it is sounded. Some people slur it almost to the vanishing point, and others make it very strong. It is especially apt to be slurred before consonants (as in "farm") and

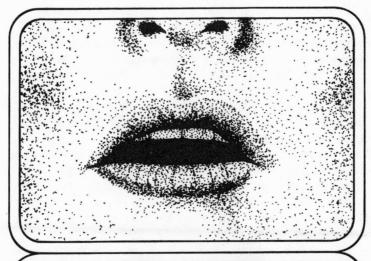

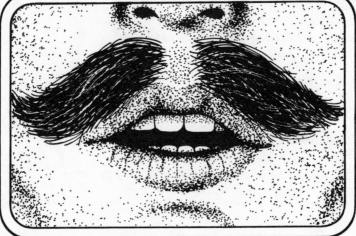

Position Eighth

in final unaccented syllables (as in "farme*r*"), and when so slurred it shows no facial position whatever. Thus "farmer" may show the positions *lt-wi-ep-ls-el-ep*, or the positions *lt-wi-ls-el*, according to the strength with which the *r* is pronounced.

4. The word "are" spoken alone by itself will show the positions *wi-ep*. But in a sentence, "are," being an auxiliary verb, and usually unstressed, becomes the equivalent of an unaccented syllable. The "wide" mouth then becomes the elliptical" mouth, as though we said not, "how *are* you?" but "*How* ur *you?*" and then the word shows the positions *el-ep*, or if the *r* be slurred, the word will show just the one position, *el*.

5. Though Position Eighth is more or less similar to Position Seventh, the two are rarely confused, inasmuch as Position Seventh is for vowel sounds and Position Eighth for a consonant sound.

6. There is a tendency, however, because of the "pucker" for the *r*, to confuse this "elliptical-puckered" (*ep*) position with the "small-oval" (*so*) position for *w* and *wh*. It will be well, therefore, to contrast the two positions as follows:

reap = *ep-na-ls*	roof	reeve
weep = *so-na-ls*	woof	weave

Summary of Position Eighth:
>   *The sound is represented by r.*
>   *The facial appearance is "elliptical puckered."*
>   *The symbol of representation is ep.*

Resolve:

reef = *ep-na-lt*	farm	verb	farmer
roof	barb	worm	firmer
room	our	free	rumor
ruff	fur	brief	reefer
rough	myrrh	prove	rubber
poor	herb	brow	poorer
arm	firm	armor	briefer

We are firm. = *so-na el-(ep)* * *lt-el-ep-ls.*
Are we? = *wi- (ep) so-na?*
A rough burr.
A poor room.
We were far.
Were *we* rough?

Resolve:

ls-ep-na-lt = brief	*ls-ep-wi-so*
so-el-ep-ls	*ls-wi-(ep)-ls*
lt-el-ep-ls	*ls-ep-pu-lt*

so-na el-(ep) lt-ep-na.
so-na so-el-(ep) ep-el-lt.
so-na so-el-(ep) lt-el-ep-ls-el-(ep).

---

*When the position *ep* is put in parenthesis, ( ) it is meant to denote that the r sound is more or less weak, and it depends upon the speaker whether it is made sufficiently strong to show its "elliptical-puckered" position.

Review of Preceding Lessons 3 and 4.

Position	Sounds	Facial Appearance	Symbol
6th-5th	ow	"wide" plus "small-oval"	*wi-so*
7th	short ŭ, u in "fur"	"elliptical" mouth	*el*
8th	r	"elliptical-puckered"	*ep*

Position Ninth *(rn)*

For the sound of accented short ĭ (as in "pit"), unaccented short ĭ (as in pulpit"), unaccented long ē (as in "believe"), and for the sound represented by the consonant *y* (as in "youth"), the lips assume a *relaxed narrow* appearance. The corners of the mouth are not drawn back and parted as in the "narrow" position for accented long ē.

REMARKS

1. Observe that the *y* in "myth," the *ie* in "sieve," etc., have the sound of short ĭ, and hence show this Position Ninth. Further, what is commonly called long ē before *r*, in such words as "fear," "weir," "here," etc., in ordinary colloquial speech has really the sound of short ĭ, and therefore shows Position Ninth, not Position First.

The sound of unaccented short ĭ, and the sound of unaccented long ē are really one and the same sound, and the sound is very close to accented short ĭ. The same sound occurs collo-

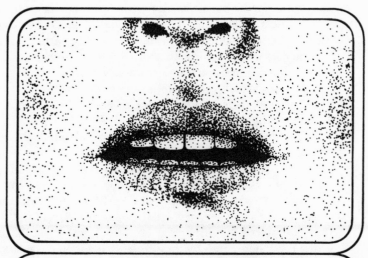

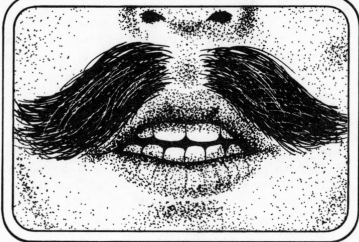

Position Ninth

quially also for an unaccented *e* in a final -ed (heated), -es (wishes), and for final unaccented *y* (happy), and hence these vowels also will show Position Ninth. The *e* in the article "the" when the next word begins with a vowel sound also has this unaccented short *ĭ* sound and shows Position Ninth.

Y is a consonant when the initial letter of a word.

2. This position is called the "relaxed-narrow" position, and is represented by the abbreviation *rn* (for "*r*elaxed-*n*arrow").

3. The unaccented *ai* in such words as "certain," the unaccented *a* in such words as "surface," "courage," the unaccented *e* in final syllables in -ent (statement) and -ence (presence) —all vary in sound according to the speaker between unaccented short *ĭ* (when they will show Position Ninth, *rn*) and unaccented short *ŭ* (when they will show Position Seventh, *el*).

4. To observe the distinction between Position Ninth and Position First, note carefully the difference between the position occurring for the unaccented *e* in "prefer" (*ls-ep-rn-lt-el-(ep)*) and for the accented long *ē* in "briefer" (*ls-ep-na-lt-el-(ep)*).

5. A further contrast of the "narrow" (*na*) and "relaxed-narrow" (*rn*) positions, as in the following contrast of accented long *ē* and accented short *ĭ*, will be valuable:

beef = *ls-na-lt*	eve	weep	reap
biff = *ls-rn-lt*	if	whip	rip

Summary of Position Ninth:

The sounds are short ĭ, unaccented long ē and consonant y.
The facial appearance is a "relaxed-narrow" mouth.
The symbol of representation is rn.

Resolve:

ye = *rn-na*	if	weir	appear
you	hip	rear	hurry
vim	imp	brim	wormy
bib	ear	primer	refer
whim	fear	river	reprove
rim	mere	hearer	revere

We are here. = *so-na el-(ep) rn-ep.*
Hurry up!
We fear him.
We free you.
You hear me?
You reprove me.
We hear a river.
We appear firmer.

Resolve:

ls-ep-rn-ls	*lt-el-ep-rn*
lt-rn-ep	*ep-rn-ls-ep-na-lt*
ls-ep-rn-lt-el-(ep)	*el-ls-rn-ep*

el ep-el-lt ls-ep-rn-ls.
el ls-ep-rn-ls ep-el-lt.
so-na ep-rn-ls-ep-pu-lt rn-pu. *
so-na ls-ep-rn-lt-el-(ep) el lt-el-ep-rn ls-el-lt.

---

*The word "you" when correctly pronounced will show the positions as
indicated. The word is very commonly slurred, however, according to the
speaker, all the way through "y00" (*rn-so*) to "yer" (*rn-el-(ep)*). But it has been
deemed best throughout the symbols in this book to keep the analysis of "you"
uniform as in the text above, (*rn-pu*).

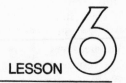

Review of Preceding Lessons 4 and 5

Position	Sounds	Facial Appearance	Symbol
8th	r	"elliptical-puckered"	*ep*
9th	short ĭ, unaccented		
	long ē, consonant y	"relaxed-narrow"	*rn*

The diphthongal sound of long *u* (as in "mute") is a combination of *y* and long $\overline{oo}$, thus, y$\overline{oo}$ = long *ū*. Therefore the positions shown by the sound of the long *u* are a combination of the ninth and fourth, that is, of the "relaxed-narrow" (*rn*) and the "puckered" (*pu*) positions. This combination is represented by a combination of the symbols, thus, *rn-pu*.

REMARKS

1. It will be found that before *r*, long *ū* is a combination not of *y* and long *oo*, but of *y* and short *ŏŏ*, thus showing the combination *rn-so*. Thus, the word "pure" is not *ls-rn-pu-ep*, but is *ls-rn-so-ep*.

2. Unaccented long *u* (as in "voluble") also shows the combination *rn-so*, and not *rn-pu*.

Resolve:

few = *lt-rn-pu*	fume	puma	pure
view	pew	review	fury

Resolve:

lt-rn-pu-ls   *ls-rn-pu*
ls-rn-pu-ls-el   *ep-rn-lt-rn-pu*

The diphthongal sound of long $\bar{\imath}$ (as in "high") shows a combination of Positions Sixth and Ninth, that is, of the "wide" (*wi*) and the "relaxed-narrow" (*n*) positions. This combination is represented by a combination of the symbols, thus, *wi-rn*.

Resolve:

high = *wi-rn*	pipe	ire	ripe
fie	why	fire	rife
fife	wife	pyre	rhyme
buy	wipe	rye	ivy

Resolve:

lt-wi-rn-lt	*ep-wi-rn-ls*
so-wi-rn-ep	*ls-wi-rn-ls*
wi-rn-ep	*wi-rn-lt-rn*

REMARKS

Unaccented long $\bar{\imath}$ (as in "gigantic") shows a combination of Positions Seventh and Ninth, that is of the "elliptical" (*el*) and the "relaxed-narrow" (*rn*). This combination is represented by a combination of the symbols, thus, *el-rn*.

This unaccented long *i* sound is very common in the two words "by" and "my" when these words occur unstressed in a sentence. When stressed, however, these words show the regular positions for long $\bar{\imath}$, namely, *wi-rn*. This will all be clear if the words "my mitt" be spoken, emphasizing first the word "my," when it will show the positions *ls-wi-rn*; and then repeating the words and this time emphasizing only the word "mitt," whereupon, the word "my," being unemphasized, will show positions *ls-el-rn*.

General Summary of Position Ninth:
Short $\breve{\imath}$, unaccented long $\bar{e}$, and consonant y = "relaxed-narrow" = rn.
Long $\bar{u}$ = "relaxed-narrow" plus "puckered" = rn-pu.
Long $\bar{u}$ before r, and unaccented long $\bar{u}$ = "relaxed-narrow" plus "small-oval" = rn-so.
Long i = "wide" plus "relaxed-narrow" = wi-rn.
Unaccented long i = "elliptical" plus "relaxed-narrow" = el-rn.

Resolve:

Why are you here? = *so-wi-rn el-(ep) rn-pu rn-ep?*
You were few.
You are high.
You reprove me.
Rub my pipe.
Buy my ivy.
Buy me a broom.
I wipe my brow.
We review.
We view a river.
We were by a river.
Why move my muff?

Resolve:

rn-pu el-(ep) lt-ep-na.
wi-rn ls-wi-rn el lt-wi-(ep)-ls.
rn-pu el-ep el lt-wi-(ep)-ls-el-(ep).
rn-pu el-ep el lt-wi-rn-lt-el-(ep).
wi-rn ls-pu-lt ls-el-rn lt-wi-rn-lt.
rn-pu el-(ep) ls-wi-rn el ep-rn-lt-el-(ep).

Review of Preceding Lessons 5 and 6

Position	Sounds	Facial Appearance	Symbol
9th	short ĭ, unaccented long ē, consonant y	"relaxed-narrow"	rn
9th-4th	long ū	"relaxed-narrow" plus "puckered"	rn-pu
9th-5th	long ū before r, and unaccented long ū	"relaxed-narrow" plus "small-oval"	rn-so
6th-9th	long ī	"wide" plus "relaxed-narrow"	wi-rn
7th-9th	unaccented long ī	"elliptical" plus "relaxed-narrow"	el-rn

Position Tenth (tf)

For the sounds represented by the letters *th* (as in "thin" and "then") the *front* of the *tongue* is visible between the teeth.

REMARKS

1. The general shape of the lips for this position is similar to Position Seventh, the "elliptical" (*el*) position.

2. This position is called the "tongue-front" position, and is represented by the abbreviation *tf* (for "tongue-front").

Summary of Position Tenth:

The sound is represented by th.
The facial appearance is "tongue-front."
The symbol of representation is tf.

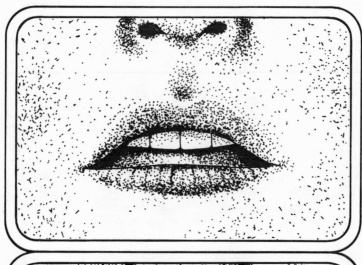

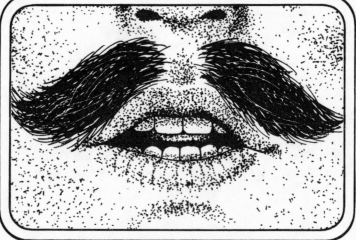

Position Tenth

Resolve:

thee = *tf-na*	thew	thigh	Ruth
thou	through	myth	youth
thumb	thrive	earth	wither

Resolve:

so-rn-tf   *lt-rn-lt-tf*
tf-ep-na   *ls-el-tf-el-(ep)*

ls-wi-rn tf-el lt-wi-(ep)-ls.
rn-pu el-(ep) ls-el-rn ls-ep-el-tf-el-(ep).

Position Eleventh *(tg)*

For the sounds represented by the letters *t* (as in "time"), *d* (as in "dime"), and *n* (as in "nine"), the *tongue* touches the upper *gum*; while the lips are in the same position as Position Ninth, the "relaxed-narrow" (*rn*) position.

REMARKS

1. This position is called the "tongue-to-gum" position, and is represented by the abbreviation *tg* (for "tongue-to-gum").

2. At the end of a word spoken alone by itself, *n* will show a slight difference from *t* and *d*, in that for *n* the tongue remains touching the upper gum, while for *t* and *d* it is brought down immediately from the upper gum. But at the beginning of a word, or in the middle of a word, or at the end of a word which stands in the middle of a sentence, the tongue naturally is brought down from the upper gum immediately after an *n* sound for forming the following sound, so that *t*, *d*, and *n* will all show precisely the same position.

3. When a *t* or a *d* follows an *n* (as in "round") the "time-element" enters into the position and is represented according to rule by the plus sign (+). If the three sounds, *t*, *d* and *n*, come together (as in "didn't"), they are written *tg* + *tg*.

4. As the lips in this position are the same as in the "relaxed-

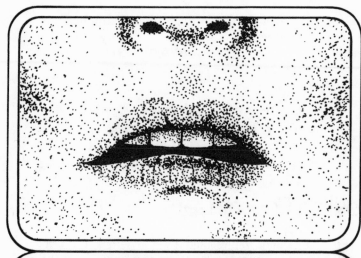

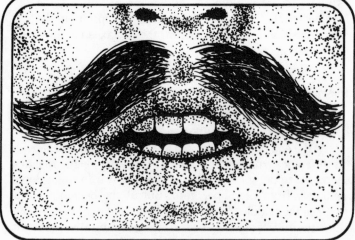

Position Eleventh

narrow," it will be found valuable to contrast the two positions
as follows, noting the change in the tongue. Contrast:

| ye = *rn-na* | year | yard | tooth |
| tea = *tg-na* | near | nard | youth |

Summary of Position Eleventh:
>   *The sounds are represented by t, d, n.*
>   *The facial appearance is "tongue-to-gum."*
>   *The symbol of representation is tg.*

Resolve:

knee = *tg-na*	truth	feet	deprive
tooth	try	pout	derive
twine	drum	fruit	buffoon
tar	tiff	put	thirteen
down	hear	art	mutton
nerve	new	hurt	diner
dream	time	rift	dinner

> We were in the yard = *so-na so-el-(ep) rn-tg*
>   *tf-el rn-wi-(ep)-tg.*
> We were near the farm.
> We dive in the river.
> I referred him to* you.
> Do* you eat fruit?
> How do* you do?
> Did you write it?
> Did you eat the tough beef?
> Did the diver find the diamond?
> Didn't you hear me?
> Didn't we buy a ton?
> The tree dipped with dew.
> Tie the ribbon tight.
> Drive me near the tomb.
> Buy me a new typewriter.
> We heard you were in an apartment.

---

*See remark 6, Position Fifth.

Resolve:

lt-el-ep-tg	*ls-wi-rn-tg*
tg-el-ep-ls	*tg-ep-wi-rn-ls*
so-na-tg	*tg-ep-pu-ls-el-(ep)*

wi-rn el-ep-tg ls-el-rn tf-el-ls.
tg-rn-tg rn-pu rn-ep tf-el tg-ep-el-ls?
tg-rn-tg tf-el tf-na-lt ep-el-tg lt-wi-(ep)?
so-na el-(ep) tf-ep-pu so-rn-tf tg-rn-tg-el-(ep).
wi-rn tg-rn-tg + tg tg-ep-na-ls rn-pu so-el-(ep) rn-ep.

Review of Preceding Lessons 6 and 7

Position	Sounds	Facial Appearance	Symbol
9th-4th	long ū	"relaxed-narrow" plus "puckered"	*rn-pu*
9th-5th	long ū before r, and unaccented long ū.	"relaxed-narrow" plus "small-oval"	*rn-so*
6th-9th	long ī	"wide" plus "relaxed-narrow"	*wi-rn*
7th-9th	unaccented long ī	"elliptical" plus "relaxed-narrow"	*el-rn*
10th	th	"tongue-front"	*tf*
11th	t, d, n	"tongue-to-gum"	*tg*

Position Twelfth *(ag)*

For the sound represented by the letter *l* (as in "leaf"), the *apex*, or point, only of the tongue touches the upper *gum*; while the lips are the same as for Position Seventh, the "elliptical" (*el*) position.

REMARKS

1. This position is called the "apex-to-gum" position, and is represented by the abbreviation *ag* (for "apex-to-gum").

2. This position is sometimes confused with the preceding "tongue-to-gum" (tg) position for *t, d,* and *n.* It differs from the "tongue-to-gum" position, however, in two essentials, namely, (a) that in this "apex-to-gum" position only the apex or point of the tongue touches the upper gum, while in the "tongue-to-

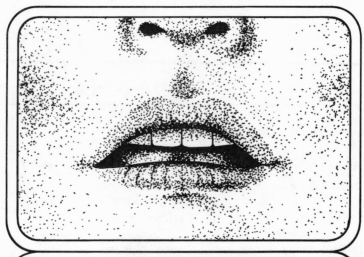

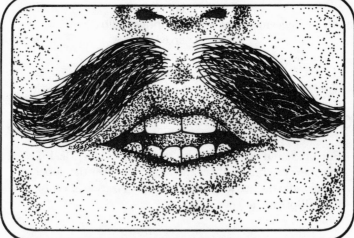

Position Twelfth

gum" position the whole front part of the tongue touches the upper gum; and (b) that in this "apex-to-gum" position the lips have the "elliptical" shape, while in the "tongue-to-gum" position the lips have the "relaxed-narrow" shape. Thus the lips are further parted for *l* than for *t*, *d*, and *n*. With the above points in mind, contrast the following:

tea = *tg-na*	dude	time	meat	food
lea = *ag-na*	lute	lime	meal	fool
noon	turn	hut	burn	white
loon	learn	hull	pearl	while

Summary of Position Twelfth:

> The sound is represented by l.
> The facial appearance is "apex-to-gum."
> The symbol of representation is ag.

Resolve:

leaf = *ag-na-lt*	leer	owl	parlor
leap	lute	hull	evil
loop	life	lull	people
lard	peal	hurl	Bible
loud	tool	pearl	idle
love	rule	fill	pupil
lump	full	file	funeral
learn	pull	miller	interval
lip	mari	ruler	liberal

Will you dine with me? = *so-rn-ag rn-pu tg-wi-rn-tg so-rn-tf ls-na*?
We will rule a line.
We will leap a river.
We will light the light.
You will learn the evil.
Will you turn a new leaf?
We'll leave you with Peter.
We'll fill the parlor with light.
You're in my light.

I've done my duty.
I've learned the rule.
I'll be with you in the interval.
The worm will turn.
Do you hear the loud drum?
My brother will need the tool.
Did you "loop the loop"?
Did you file the wire in two?
Did you hear the murmur in the lull?
I'll trouble you to leave the room.
You will find me in the field near the fir tree.

Resolve:

lt-na-ag-tg	*so-wi-rn-ag-tg*
tg-el-+ls-ag	*ls-rn-ag-na-lt*
tg-el-el-ls-ag	*tf-rn-ag*
ag-rn-lt-el-(ep)	*ls-rn-pu-ag*

tf-el tg-pu-ag so-rn-ag el-ep-tg rn-pu.
wi-rn so-rn-ag ls-so-ag rn-pu wi-so-tg.
so-na-ag ep-el-tg tg-so tf-el lt-na-ag-tg.
tg-so rn-pu lt-wi-rn-+tg ls-na el tg-el-ag ls-rn-pu-ls-rn-ag?
wi-rn so-rn-ag ag-na-lt tf-el so-na-ag rn-tg tf-el ls-wi-(ep)-tg.
rn-pu so-rn-ag lt-wi-rn-+tg ls-na rn-tg tf-el ls-wi-(ep)-ag-el-(ep).
tf-el ls-el-+tg (mutton = mutt'n) rn-pu so-rn-ag lt-wi-rn-+tg
   tg-el-lt, ls-el-tg so-na-ag na-tg tf-el lt-ep-pu-tg.

Review of Preceding Lessons 7 and 8

Position	Sounds	Facial Appearance	Symbol
10th	th	"tongue-front"	*tf*
11th	t, d, n	"tongue-to-gum"	*tg*
12th	l	"apex-to-gum"	*ag*

Position Thirteenth *(st)*

For the sound of broad *a* (as in "all") and for the sound of the *o* in "for," "form," etc., the lips are open in the shape of a *spherical triangle.*

REMARKS

1. Observe that this broad *a* sound occurs also for the letters *aw* (as in "awl"), *au* (as in "sauce"), *ou* (as in "bought"), *oa* (as in "broad"), etc., and hence all these vowels, having the same sound as broad *a*, show the same position as broad *a*.

2. This position is called the "spherical-triangle" position, and is represented by the abbreviation *st* (for "spherical-triangle").

3. It was stated in remark 4, Position Sixth, that short *ŏ* (as in "odd") was sometimes heard as an extreme short sound of Italian *a* (*ah*), and sometimes as an extreme short sound of broad *a* (*aw*). In the former case, short *ŏ* will show the "wide" (*wi*) position, and in the latter case it will show the "spherical-triangle" (*st*) position. In the symbols in this book short *ŏ* is usually represented as giving the "wide" (*wi*) position inasmuch

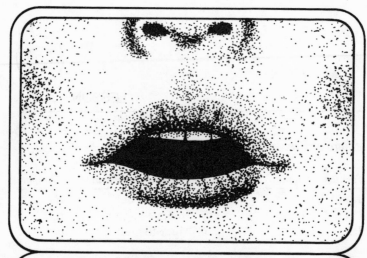

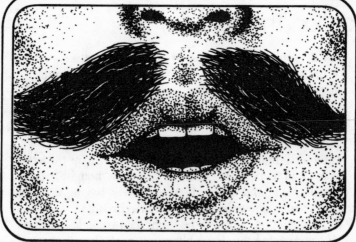

Position Thirteenth

as this position is a little more common. But pupils in their mirror practice must be guided by their own pronunciation.

4. The sound of the *o* in "of" and "from" is correctly short ŏ, showing, according to the speaker, either the "wide" (*wi*) or the "spherical-triangle" (*st*) position. But colloquially the *o* in "of" and "from" is heard as the equivalent of an unaccented short ŭ sound, as though the words were "uv" and "frum," showing the "elliptical" (*el*) position. This is the position which will usually be indicated for the *o* sound in these words in this book.

5. There is a slight tendency to confuse the position for broad *a* (*st*) with that for Italian *a* (*wi*). It will be valuable, therefore, to contrast the two as follows, noting, (a) that the mouth is opened more widely for Italian *a* than for broad *a*, and (b) that the corners of the lips are farther apart for Italian *a* than for broad *a*. Contrast:

far = *lt-wi-ep*   farm   barn
for = *lt-st-ep*   form   born

6. The sound of the *o* before *r* (as in "more") will, as a rule in ordinary speech, show this "spherical-triangle" (*st*) position, even though the sound is not *aw*. Similarly also *oo* in "door," *ou* in "four," etc., having the same sound as the *o* in "more" will show the "spherical-triangle" position. However, by not a few people this sound of *o* in "more" is made like the long ō sound in "go," and then shows the same position as long ō. Therefore, words like "more," "door," etc., will not enter into the practice words and sentences until long ō has been described.

Summary of Position Thirteenth:
    The sounds are broad a (aw) and o in "form."
    The facial appearance is a "spherical-triangle."
    The symbol of abbreviation is st.

Resolve:

fall = *lt-st-ag*	thaw	ought	forlorn
ball	thought	pawn	laurel
bought	thorn	dawn	deform
born	daw	lawn	reward
warm	gnaw	author	abroad
worn	law	lawyer	applaud
wharf	vault	former	defraud
raw	orb	reform	default
yawl	warn	perform	withdraw

You will mind the law = *rn-pu so-rn-ag ls-wi-rn + tg tf-el ag-st.*
   I moved my pawn.
   I've been abroad all winter.
   I've the money in the vault.
   Were you born in London (*ag-el-tg + tg*)?
   The people will applaud you.
   I'll draw the thorn from your thumb.
   I'll leave my bond in default of the money.
   Be alert, or he will defraud you.
   You will find the ball in the other yard.
   I thought you were the author of the law.
   The thaw will fill the pond with water.
   The typewriter will be bought by my brother.
   A broad-minded lawyer will not admit defeat.
   You will feel forlorn if we all withdraw.
   The laurel tree will fall with a high wind.
   The knife I bought, he imported from Berlin.
   If you will not report me, I will reward you.
   I'll report you if you do not perform your duty.
   I've offered a reward for the return of the diamond.
   The ball will rebound to you from the wall.

Resolve:

so-st-ag	*tg-st-ag*
ls-ep-st-ag	*lt-st-(ep)-ls-el-ag*
tf-ep-st-ag	*st-ls-el-(ep)-tg*
ag-st-(ep)-tg	*tg-st-(ep)-ls-el-ag*

wi-rn ls-st-tg tf-el lt-wi-(ep)-ls.
wi-rn-lt ls-st-tg tf-el ls-el-ep-ag.
so-na so-rn-ag ag-rn-lt el-ls-ep-st-tg lt-st-ep el + rn-ep.
so-na so-rn-ag so-rn-tf-tg-ep-st lt-ep-el-ls tf-el lt-na-ag-tg.
tf-rn st-tf-el-(ep) so-rn-ag ls-rn (be) rn-ep rn-tg tf-el lt-st-ag.
na tg-rn-tg tg-wi-tg ep-rn-so-st-(ep)-tg ls-na so-rn-tf ls-el-tg-rn.
rn-lt wi-rn lt-st-ag, tf-el lt-st-ag-tg so-rn-ag tg-wi-tg ls-rn
   ls-wi-rn-tg.
so-rn-tf-wi-so-tg tg-wi-so-tg so-na so-rn-ag st-ag ls-rn rn-ep
   lt-st-ep el ls-el-tg-tf.

The dipthongal sound of *oy* (as in "toy") shows a combination of Positions Thirteenth and Ninth, that is, of the "spherical-triangle" (*st*) and the "relaxed-narrow" (*rn*) positions. Combination of the symbols, thus *st-rn.*

REMARKS

The sound of *oy* is common also for the letters *oi* (as in "oil"), which show, therefore, the same combination of positions as *oy*.

Resolve:

void = *lt-st-rn-tg*	toil	devoid
boy	loin	alloy
roil	oil	annoy
broil	avoid	loyal

Resolve:

st-rn-ag	*lt-st-rn-ag*
ls-st-rn-ag-el-(ep)	*lt-st-rn-ls-ag*

General Summary of Position Thirteenth:
   Broad a (aw) and o in "form" = "spherical-triangle" = st.
   oy = "spherical-triangle" plus "relaxed-narrow" = st-rn.

Review of Preceding Lessons 8 and 9

Position	Sounds	Facial Appearance	Symbol
12th	l	"apex-to-gum"	*ag*
13th	broad a (aw), and o in "form"	"spherical-triangle"	*st*
13th-9th	oy	"spherical-triangle" plus "relaxed-narrow"	*st-rn*

Position Fourteenth *(tn)*

For the sounds represented by the letters *s* (as in "see") and *z* (as in "zebra"), the lips show a *narrow* opening, with the muscles at the corners of the mouth slightly *tightened* or strained.

REMARKS

1. Observe that soft *c* (as in "piece") has the sound of *s*, and hence shows this Position Fourteenth.

2. This position is called the "tightened-narrow" position, and is represented by the abbreviation *tn* (for "tightened-narrow").

3. This position is not a little like Position First, the "narrow" position, but the two are almost never confused, inasmuch as the "narrow" position covers a vowel sound and the "tightened narrow" covers consonant sounds. It may be noted, however, in addition to the "tightening," that the teeth are closer together for *s* and *z* than for long $\bar{e}$.

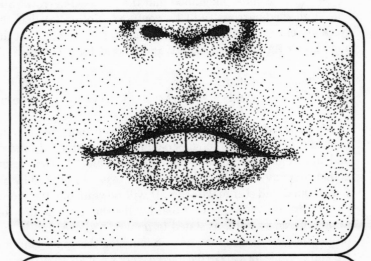

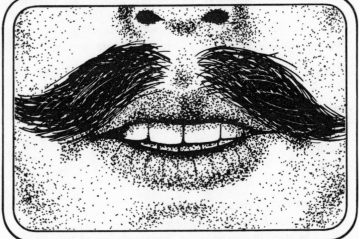

Position Fourteenth

4. There is more likelihood that the "relaxed-narrow" and the "tightened-narrow" will be confused. Noting (a) that the teeth are closer together for *s* and *z* than for *y*, and (b) that the muscles are tightened for *s* and *z*, and relaxed for *y*, contrast:

see = *tn-na*	sealed	sot	saw	sooth
ye = *rn-na*	yield	yacht	yaw	youth

5. In rapid, natural speech there is even more liability to confusion between the "tongue-to-gum" position (for *t*, *d*, and *n*) and this "tightened-narrow" position (for *s* and *z*). The reason is that in many words a *t*, *d*, or *n* sound may be replaced by an *s* or *z* sound and still make sense. It will be valuable, therefore, to contrast as follows, noting that for the shape of the lips the same differences hold, as stated in remark 4 above, and in addition, that the tongue may be seen touching the upper gum for *t*, *d* and *n*, while for *s* and *z* the tongue is not see at all. Contrast:

sop = *tn-wi-ls*	swine	soil	mice
top = *tg-wi-ls*	twine	toil	mite
son	sigh	wars	pause
ton	tie	wart	brought
surf	sue	peace	toys
turf	dew	peet	toyed
sooth	saw	muss	moose
tooth	daw	mud	moot

Summary of Position Fourteenth:
   The sounds are represented by s and z.
   The facial appearance is a "tightened-narrow" mouth.
   The symbol of representation is tn.

Resolve:

sea = *tn-na*	soil	bus	mister
sooth	sphere	purse	sister
soot	spear	miss	wisdom
psalm	sweet	use	arise

south	sly	mice	revise
sup	snarl	laws	surmise
serve	strive	toys	suffice
sip	peace	applause	despise
sue	moose	because	scissors
sigh	puss	advice	otherwise
saw	house	whisper	supervise

The sea is smooth = *tf-el tn-na rn-tn tn-ls-pu-tf*.

    Is the steamer due?

    Is the storm severe?

    Is business prosperous?

    Was the surmise right?

    The boy is on the street.

    The lawyer hasn't seen me.

    The boy is with his brother.

    I'll apprise you of the time.

    A sordid life is a false life.

    I lost a dollar from my purse.

    Did you find the scissors for me?

    I'll offer a prize if you'll try.

    We must arise with the rising sun.

    The lawyer will preside with wisdom.

    We will serve turtle soup for dinner.

    The farm is on the Mississippi River.

    The blotter is spoiled for further use.

    It'll be wise if you will do otherwise.

    His brother is in love with my sister.

    Behind all business is the typewriter.

    The mystery of life is too deep to solve.

    The boy was delighted with his new toys.

    I'll promise to do it soon, if possible.

    The minister will read the fifteenth psalm.

    Did you find the deepest part of the stream?

    You must sweep out the lawyer's office for him.

    I will write to you about the first of the month.

    If we've seen Boston, we've seen the Hub of the Universe.

Resolve:

tn-el-ls	*tn-rn- + ls-ag*
ls-ep-na-tn	*so-el-ep-tn-tg*
tg-el-tn-tg	*lt-rn-tn-rn-tg*
tn-wi-rn-tn	*tn-rn-lt-rn-ep*

so-el-tg tg-wi-rn-ls rn-tn rn-tg?
tf-el tg-ep-pu-tf rn-tn rn-tg-el-ep-tg-el-ag.
tf-el ls-ep-wi-rn-tn rn-tn tg-pu tn-ls-st-ag.
tg-rn-tg rn-pu rn-ep tf-el so-rn-tn-ls-el-(ep)?
tf-el tg-el-tn-tg so-rn-ag el-ep-tg ls-el-rn wi-rn-tn.
tg-wi-rn-ls so-rn-ag ls-ep-pu-lt ls-el-rn so-rn-tn-tg-el-ls.
wi-rn rn-ep el ls-el-ep-ls-el-(ep) rn-tg tf-el tg-ep-na-tg-wi-ls-tn.
tf-el ls-wi-rn-tn-el-(ep) st-(ep)-tg-tn rn-tn ls-el-tg-rn rn-tg tf-el
    lt-st-ag-tg.
tn-so-na-tg el-(ep) tf-el rn-pu-tn-rn-tn el-lt el-tg-lt-el-ep-tn-rn-tg-rn.
tg-rn-tg tf-el st-(ep)-tn ep-el-tg tf-el ls-wi-rn-ag rn-tg tg-pu
    ls-rn-tg-rn-tg-tn?

Review of Preceding Lessons 9 and 10

Position	Sounds	Facial Appearance	Symbol
13th	broad a (aw), and o in "form"	"spherical-triangle"	*st*
13th-9th	oy	"spherical-triangle" + "relaxed-narrow"	*st-rn*
14th	s, z	"tightened-narrow"	*tn*

The dipthongal sound of long ō (as in "go") shows a combination of Positions Thirteenth and Fifth, that is, of the "spherical-triangle" (*st*) and "small-oval" (*so*) positions. This is represented by a combination of the symbols, thus, *st-so*.

REMARKS

1. The letters *au* in "hautboy," *eau* in "beau," *eo* in "yeoman," *ew* in "sew," *oa* in "roam," *ou* in "shoulder," and *ow* in "grow,"—all have the same sound as long ō, and hence show the same combination of positions, namely, *st-so*.

2. In rapid, natural speech, long ō before *r* (as in "more") slurs off the final "small-oval" (*so*) position usually seen in long ō, leaving only the "spherical-triangle" (*st*) position. This is the *o* before *r* spoken of in remark 6, Position Thirteenth. However, some careful speakers keep the "small-oval" before *r* even in rapid speech; hence the pupil in mirror practice must be guided by his own pronunciation.

3. In rapid, natural speech again, unaccented long ō (as in "violin") also slurs off the "small-oval" (*so*) position, leaving only the "spherical-triangle" (*st*) position. Not infrequently, also, this unaccented *o* is still further slurred and is heard as the equivalent of unaccented short *u*, thus showing the "elliptical" (*el*) position.

4. Occasionally, though not often, long $\bar{o}$ is spoken by some people without a dipthongal sound, but with a sound approximating short $\breve{o}\breve{o}$ (the word "wholly" is most frequently so heard) and showing thus just the "small-oval" (so) position.

5. Long $\bar{o}$ (st-so) is sometimes confused with ow (wi-so). It will be of service, therefore, to contrast the two sounds as follows, noting that though they both end with the same position, long $\bar{o}$ begins with the "spherical-triangle" (st) position, while ow begins with the "wide" (wi) position. Contrast:

tone = tg-st-so-tg	vote	slow	blow	load
town = tg-wi-so-tg	vowed	slough	plough	loud

General Summary:

Long $\bar{o}$ = "spherical-triangle" plus "small-oval" = st-so.

Resolve:

foam = lt-st-so-ls	low	ode	willow
boat	so	hole	sorrow
woe	loaf	hose	tomorrow
roe	hope	devote	propose
though	oath	widow	promote

How will you know the truth? = *wi-so so-rn-ag rn-pu tg-st-so tf-el tg-ep-pu-tf?*
I want to know all.
The wind blows fiercely.
Will I see you tomorrow?
I heard the news by 'phone.
I sincerely hope you are right.
I was about to propose it to you.
The woman will no doubt believe me.
Your new idea will promote business.
I hope you will find room for us all.
I hope three or four more will be enough.
I would be proud to own the house.
The boy was delighted with his willow whistle.
He devotes his life to his invalid mother.
Sow the wind, and (*el-* + *tg*) reap the whirlwind.

the water poured over the side of the boat.
Won't you drive me around the town?
Won't you darn the hole in my hose?
I don't propose to submit to it.
Don't allow him to impose upon you.
Don't whisper so loud or others will hear.
You'll lose the trolley if you don't hurry.
You will rouse the house if you don't lower your voice.

Resolve:

ep-st-so-ls   ls-ag-st-so
lt-ag-st-so   tf-ep-st-so

so-na el-(ep) ls-ep-wi-so-tg tg-so tg-st-so rn-pu.
so-na so-rn-ag el-ep-wi-rn-lt ls-el-rn ls-st-so-tg.
wi-rn ep-st-so-tg rn-pu wi-rn + so-tg tg-wi-tg ls-rn rn-ep.
so-el-(ep) rn-pu tf-rn st-tf-el-ep) el-lt tf-el ls-st-so-rn-ls?
wi-rn lt-rn-ep tf-el ep-st-so-ls so-rn-ag tg-wi-tg st-so-ag-tg el-tn.
tg-rn-tg rn-pu lt-st-so-tg lt-st-(ep) tf-rn st-ag-tg-el-(ep)-ls-el-tg?
wi-rn so-el-tn el-ls-wi-so-tg tf-ep-na ls-wi-rn-ag-tn lt-wi-(ep)-tf-el-
        (ep) st-lt.

Review of Preceding Lessons 10 and 11

Position	Sounds	Facial Appearance	Symbol
14th	s,z	"tightened-narrow"	*tn*
13th-5th	long ō	"spherical-triangle" plus "small-oval"	*st-so*

Position Fifteenth *(lo)*

For the sound of accented short ă (as in "mat"), the lips assume the position of a *large oval*, the corners of the upper lip being slightly drawn upward.

REMARKS

1. A valuable aid in recognizing this position, when there is a good light on the face, will be found in the forward position of the tongue just barely touching the lower teeth.

2. This position is called the "large-oval" position, and is represented by the abbreviation *lo* (for "*large-oval*").

3. The *a* in such words as "pass," "last," "ask," etc., is most commonly heard, though with technical inaccuracy, with this short ă sound. For the *a* in such words in the symbols in this book the representation *lo* will therefore be used to designate its most common facial appearance. But pupils in their mirror practice must be guided by their own pronunciation.

4. The unaccented *a* in such words as "appoint" is not short ă, but colloquially has the sound of unaccented short ŭ, thus showing the "elliptical" (*el*) position, as stated in remark 2, Position Seventh.

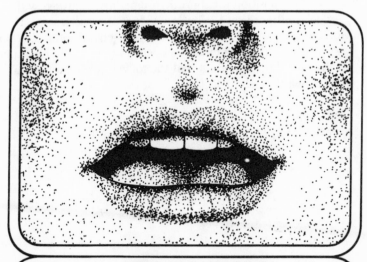

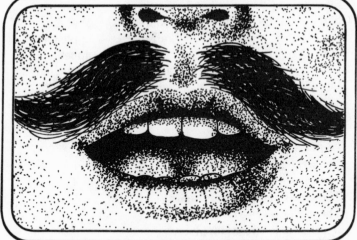

Position Fifteenth

5. This position for short ă is sometimes confused with the "wide" (*wi*) position for Italian *a*. It will be of service, therefore, to contrast the two sounds and positions, as follows, noting especially (a) that the mouth is opened more widely for Italian *a* than for short ă, and (b) that the tongue is back for Italian *a*, and forward for short ă.

hat = *lo-tg*	pan	mat	pat
heart = *wi-(ep)-tg*	barn	mart	part

Summary of Position Fifteenth:
>   The sound is short ă.
>   The facial appearance is a "large-oval."
>   The symbol of representation is lo.

Resolve:

fat = *lt-lo-tg*	lap	battle	animal
bat	sap	ramble	abandon
rap	ram	raffle	apple-pie
yam	as	dabster	appetite
that	family	admirable	dandelion
tap	palate	labyrinth	depravity

The battle will be lost. = *tf-el ls-lo-tg-ag so-rn-ag
     ls-rn ag-st-tn-tg.*
I will use a bamboo pole.
The wrap is not warm enough.
Did you slip on the banana peel?
The sand filtered into my boots.
The trolley service is admirable.
It is useless to oppose his plans.
The time appointed is now far past.
Have you an appetite for apple-pie?
Who planted that idea in your mind?
I will try to adapt my plan to yours.
We demand that you allow us more time.
While you have life, do not abandon hope.
I *will* learn to understand with the eyes.
The batsman hit the ball for a home run.

Don't pronounce your words so rapidly.
The hammer dropped upon the man's foot.
The busiest street in town is Wall Street.
He plans to be married in the summer time.
We've planned to have a reunion of our class.
Some time must elapse before he will return.
We were at the dance till the "wee sma' hours."
I've dabbled with art, but I'm not a dabster.
I still hope the matter will turn out all right.
He had improved, but on Tuesday he had a relapse.
Happily we didn't know of it until it was all over.
The farmer foretold that we would have a bad thunderstorm.

Resolve:

ls-ag-lo-tg	*lo-ls-ag*
tn-ls-lo-tg	*ls-ep-lo-+ls-ag*
tn-tg-lo-+ls	*ls-el-tg-lo-tg-el*
tg-ep-lo-+ls	*tn-lo-+ls-ag*

rn-pu el-ep el-tg lo-ls-tg ls-rn-pu-ls-rn-ag.
so-na so-rn-ag tn-ls-lo-tg tf-el ep-rn-lt-el-(ep).
tf-el ls-lo-tg tg-rn-tg+tg lo-lt tf-el lo-ls-el-(ep).
rn-so-ep lo-ls-rn-tg-wi-rn-tg rn-tn rn-+ls-ep-pu-lt-tg.
tf-el tg-ep-na rn-tn st-ag ls-st-rn-tn-tg so-rn-tf tn-lo-ls.
wi-rn tg-rn-tg+tg tg-ep-na-ls rn-pu +so-tg tg-pu tf-lo-tg.
so-el(ep) rn-pu ag-st-tn-tg rn-tg tf-el ag-lo-ls-el-ep-rn-tg-tf?
tg-rn-tg rn-pu ep-lo-ls wi-tg tf-el tg-st-ep ls-rn-lt-st-(ep)-lo-+tg?
wi-rn tg-st-so-ag-tg el-tg lo-lt-tg-el-(ep)-tg-rn-tg-el-(ep) tn-tg-st-ep-rn.

Review of Preceding Lessons 11 and 12

Position	Sounds	Facial Appearance	Symbol
13th-5th	long ō	"spherical-triangle" plus "small oval"	st-so
15th	short ă	"large oval"	lo

Position Sixteenth *(pr)*

For the sounds represented by the letters *sh* (as in "ship"), *zh* (the *s* in "measure" has the sound of *zh*), *ch* (as in "chip"), *j* (as in "jam"), and soft *g* (as in gentle"), the mouth assumes an oval position with a *protrusion*, or thrusting forward, of the lips.

REMARKS

1. Observe that *ti* (as in "ration") and *si* (as in "pension") have the sound of *sh*, and hence show the same position as *sh*. Observe also that *tch* (as in "notch") is the same sound as *ch*, and the *t* does not show a separate "tongue-to-gum" (*tg*) position. And further, *dg* (as in "ledge") is the same sound as soft *g*, and the *d* does not show a separate "tongue-to-gum" (*tg*) position either.

2. This position is called the "protruded" position, and is represented by the abbreviation *pr* (for "*protruded*").

3. In colloquial speech the *t* in such words as "fortune," and the *d* in such words as "educate" will, with most people, show this "protruded" position.

4. The "protruded" position is one of the easiest to recog-

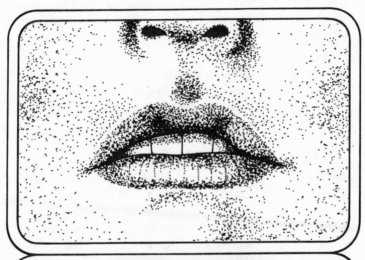

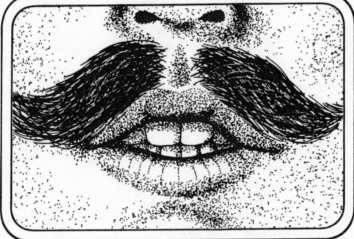

Position Sixteenth

nize, the chief difficulty being to distinguish between the number of the sounds covered. But this is a difficulty which with the context to help causes but little trouble.

Summary of Position Sixteenth:

The sounds are represented by sh, zh, ch, j and soft g.
The facial appearance is a "protruded" mouth.
The symbol of representation is pr.

Resolve:

she = *pr-na*	shine	watch	chow chow
shoot	shawl	ouch	chivalry
should	joy	harsh	chop-house
sharp	show	mush	chapter
shout	sham	merge	justice
shirt	each	wish	German
shove	huge	roach	oblige
shrive	bush	ash	orchard
ship	wash	abash	ocean

I was out in the shower = *wi-rn-so-el-tn wi-so-tg-*
    rn-tg tf-el pr-wi-so-el-(ep).
Don't touch me.
I've lost my brush.
Don't shove so hard.
I wish I knew German.
"Shine yer shoes, sir?"
The knife is not sharp.
I found the river shallow.
Will you have lunch early?
Will you have some chow chow?
We will have the hash for supper.
Did you search for the lost pin?
I wish you would be more cheerful.
Children should be seen, not heard.
We have dissolved our partnership.
The reward of perseverance is sure.
The peaches are ripe early this year.
It is a joy just to watch the ocean.

The storm did much damage in the city.
Our ideals are often beyond our reach.
My shoe is so tight it pinches my toe.
She does not wish to dance the German.
Have you been on the voyage to Bermuda?
We don't want charity; we want justice.
I've just finished the fifteenth chapter.
Don't you enjoy the study of philosophy?
Will you put the shawl over my shoulders?
We were out in the launch all the afternoon.
We've searched for the thimble high and low.
The trees in the orchard are loaded with apples.
If you'll write the note for me, I'll be much obliged.
The loss of the ship was a severe blow to our business.

Resolve:

pr-pu-tg	*tg-lo-pr*
pr-so-tg	*ls-wi-(ep)-pr*
pr-ep-wi-rn-tg	*ag-lo-pr*
lt-rn-pr	*pr-lo-tg-st-so*

so-wi-rn tg-so rn-pu pr-rn-lt-el-(ep)?
tg-rn-tg rn-pu rn-ep tf-el pr-wi-so-tg?
pr-na rn-tn el pr-wi-ls-ag-rn-lt-tg-el-(ep).
wi-rn-ag pr-st-so rn-pu tf-el tg-wi-so-tg.
wi-rn so-rn-ag ls-wi-ag-rn-pr ls-el-rn pr-pu.
wi-rn-lt el-ep-tg ls-el-rn pr-st-so-ag-tg-el-(ep).
tf-el pr-rn-ls ep-lo-tg el-ls-el-tg el pr-st-so-ag.
tf-el ls-st-rn-+ tg rn-tn-+ tg pr-wi-(ep)-ls rn-tg-el-lt.
wi-rn so-rn-pr wi-rn lo-tg el tn-tg-st-so pr-el-lt-ag.
rn-pu so-el-(ep) lt-pu-ag-rn-pr tg-wi-tg tg-so ls-rn rn-ep.

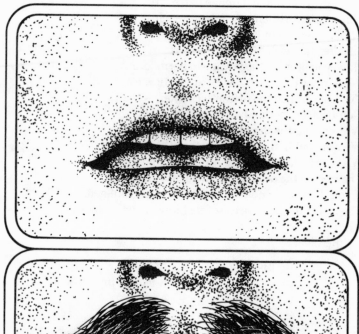

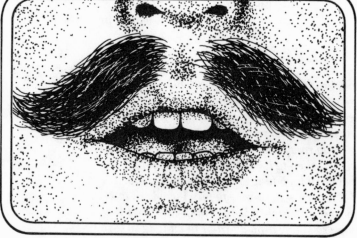

Position Seventeenth

Review of Preceding Lessons 12 and 13

Position	Sounds	Facial Appearance	Symbol
15th	short ă	"large-oval"	*lo*
16th	sh, zh, ch, j, and soft g	"protruded" mouth	*pr*

Position Seventeenth *(mo)*

For the sounds of short ĕ (as in "lĕt"), and of *a* before *r* (as in "care"), the lips assume the position of a *medium-sized oval.* The position is most like the "elliptical," but for short ĕ the corners of the mouth are further apart than for short ŭ.

REMARKS

1. Observe that *ai* in "said," *ea* in "head," and *a* in "any," have the sound of short ĕ, and hence show Position Seventeenth. Also, *ai* in "fair," and *ea* in "pear" have the sound of the *a* before *r* in "care," and hence show Position Seventh.

2. This position is called the "medium-oval" position, and is represented by the abbreviation *mo* (for "*medium-o*val").

3. It will be of service to contrast this "medium-oval" (*mo*) position for short ĕ with the "elliptical" (*el*) position for short ŭ. Note (a) that the corners of the lips are further apart for short ĕ than for short ŭ, and (b) that, if there is a good light on the face, the tongue will be seen to be forward for short ĕ and back for short ŭ. Contrast:

| bet = | *ls-mo-tg* | rest | bled |
| but = | *ls-el-tg* | rust | blood |

| dell | left | jest |
| dull | luffed | just |

4. There is also a tendency to confuse the "medium-oval" (*mo*) position for short ĕ with the "large-oval" (*lo*) position for short ă. But the mouth is open noticeably wider for the "large-oval" (*lo*) for short *a* than for the "medium-oval" (*mo*) for short ĕ.

Contrast:

| led = | *ag-mo-tg* | said | bet | red | shed | ten |
| lad = | *ag-lo-tg* | sad | bat | rat | shad | tan |

5. There is still a further tendency to confuse the "medium-oval" (*mo*) position for short ĕ with the "narrow" (*na*) position for long ē. But the lips are noticeably nearer together for long ē than for short ĕ. Contrast:

| dell = | *tg-mo-ag* | bed | said | fed |
| deal = | *tg-na-ag* | bead | seed | feed |

Summary of Position Seventeenth:

> *The sounds are short ĕ and a in "care."*
> *The facial appearance is a "medium-oval."*
> *The symbol of representation is mo.*

Resolve:

fell =	*lt-mo-ag*	sell	their	forever
bell		shell	lair	engine
well		deaf	Beth	enemy
red		leapt	wet	elephant
yell		fair	west	pleasant
theft		wear	wedge	befell
death		spare	ever	develop
left		share	sever	envelope

Did you see the sunset? = *tg-rn-tg rn-pu tn-na*
    tf-el tn-el-tg-tn-mo-tg?
Tell me what befell you.
It's no fun to be deaf.
Better be deaf than blind.
There will be a storm tomorrow.
Will you let me have an envelope?
Will you share that pear with me?
The weather last September was very wet.
You have a white elephant on your hands.
There's to be a ball at the fair tonight.
We will sell the farm for a thousand dollars.

    Resolve:

    A physician went to rent some rooms. The servant who an-
swered the bell was especially pretty. The physician wished to
know whether she was to be let with the rooms. "No," she replied, "I'm to be let alone."

    Resolve:

pr-mo-tn	*so-mo-ls*
ls-ag-mo-tn	*ep-mo-tn-tg*
tn-ls-mo-ag	*ls-mo-ep*
tn-ag-mo-ls-tg	*tn-tg-mo-ep*

wi-rn + so-tg ep-rn-tn-mo- + tg rn-tg.
tf-el ls-wi-so-el-(ep) el-lt tf-el ls-ep-mo-tn.
wi-rn tg-rn-tg + tg rn-ep so-el-tg rn-pu tn-mo-tg.
wi-rn so-rn-pr rn-pu + so-tg + tg ls-st-ag-mo-tn-tg ls-na.
so-na el-lt tn-mo-lt-el-(ep)-tg wi-so-ep lt-ep-mo- + tg-pr-rn-ls.
tf-el ls-mo-tg rn-tn ls-wi-rn-tg-rn-el-(ep) tf-el-tg tf-el tn-st-ep-tg.

    The diphthongal sound of long $\bar{a}$ (as in "$\bar{a}$le") shows a com-
bination of Positions Seventeenth and Ninth, that is, of the
"medium-oval" (*mo*), and the "relaxed-narrow" (*rn*) positions.
This combination is represented by a combination of the
symbols, thus, *mo-rn.*

REMARKS

1. The letters *ai* (as in "vain") and *ay* (as in "way") frequently have the long *ā* sound, and hence show the same combination of positions, namely, *mo-rn*.

2. Long *ā* is sometimes confused with short *ĕ*. It will be of service, therefore, to contrast the two sounds, as follows, noting especially that because of the combination of two positions for long *ā*, this sound shows a more prolonged appearance than short *ĕ*.

fell = *lt-mo-ag*	bet	let	shed	yell	stare
fail = *lt-mo-rn-ag*	bait	late	shade	Yale	stayer

3. Long *ā* (*mo-rn*) is also confused more or less with long *ī* (*wi-rn*). It will be of service, therefore, to contrast as follows, noting especially that the mouth is opened noticeably wider for long *ī* than for long *ā*.

lay = *ag-mo-rn*	say	dame	pale	rape	ways
lie = *ag-wi-rn*	sigh	dime	pile	ripe	wise

General Summary of Position Seventeenth:

short *ĕ* and *a* in "care" = "medium-oval" = mo.
long *ā* = "medium-oval" plus "relaxed-narrow" = mo-rn.

Resolve:

fay = *lt-mo-rn*	day	lathe	apron
may	lay	aid	delay
weigh	say	ale	display
ray	shay	ace	relation
yea	lave	age	newspaper
they	aim	able	favorite

It was a fine debate = *rn-tg so-el-tn el lt-wi-rn-tg tg-rn-ls-mo-rn-tg*.
I am not able to say today.
You'd better put an apron on.
I have unbounded faith in you.

How far away are the mountains.
Her favorite flower is the violet.
We'll lay the matter on the table.
Where there's a will, there's a way.
They offer a rebate on large orders.
Will you please hand me the newspaper?
I shouldn't wonder if we had some rain.
Have you ever read the "One Horse Shay"?
When they hear the news, what will they say?
It will be a favor if you will be here promptly.

Resolve:

tn-ls-ep-mo-rn	*tg-mo-rn-ls-ag*
lt-mo-rn-tf	*el-so-mo-rn*
tg-mo-rn-ls	*ls-ag-mo-rn-ls*

wi-so ls-el-pr tg-so rn-pu so-mo-rn?
tf-el tg-mo-rn ls-rn-lt-st-ep rn-mo-tn-tg-el-(ep)-tg-mo-rn.
wi-rn-ag ep-rn-ag-mo-rn-tg ls-el-rn el-tg-lt-mo-tg-pr-so-ep.
na rn-tn el wi-(ep)-tg + tg st-so-ag-tg ep-mo-ls-ep-st-ls-mo-rn-tg.
tf-el tg-mo-rn-pr-tg-tn so-rn-ag wi-(ep)-ls-rn-tg-ep-mo-rn-tg
tf-mo-ep tg-rn-tn-ls-rn-pu-tg.

Review of Preceding Lessons 13 and 14

Position	Sounds	Facial Appearance	Symbol
16th	sh, zh, ch, j, soft g	"protruded" mouth	*pr*
17th	short ĕ, a in "care"	"medium-oval"	*mo*
17th-9th	long ā	"medium-oval" plus "relaxed-narrow"	*mo-rn*

Position Eighteenth *(un)*

For the sounds represented by the letters *k* (as in "keep"), hard *g* (as in "go"), *nk* (as in "rank"), and *ng* (as in "rang"), the lips assume an open but an *undefined* position, with a tendency to approach the position of the most closely connected vowel sound.

REMARKS

1. Hard *c* (as in "can"), *ch* (as in "epoch"), *ck* (as in "back"), and *q* (as in "quaint"), all have the sound of *k*, and hence show the same position. The only effect of the *n* in *nk* and *ng* is to nasalize the following *k* and *g* sounds; the tongue does not go up to the upper gum as the pure *n* sound would require—hence the *n* shows no separate position.

2. This position is called the "undefined" position, and is represented by the abbreviation *un* (for "*un*defined").

3. The sounds of this position are all palatal sounds, and hence require no definite position of the lips; thus we have a varying lip position, approximating the position of the most closely connected sound. For example, if we say "rank," the lips

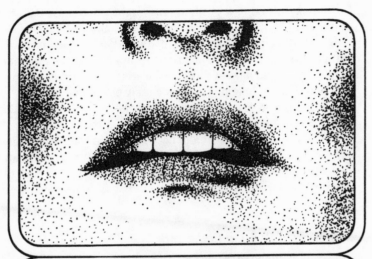

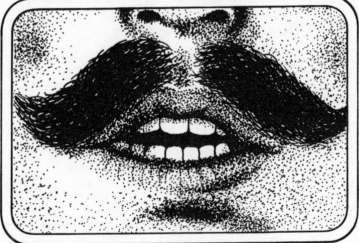

Position Eighteenth

for the *nk* will be in a position only slightly less open than the "large-oval" (*lo*) for the preceding short *ă* sound; while if we say "ink," the lips for the *nk* will be in almost the "relaxed-narrow" (*rn*) position for the preceding short *ĭ* sound. Thus these sounds, *k*, hard *g*, *nk* and *ng*, have almost the effect of a "*time-element*" or a *pause*, in prolonging the most closely connected sound.

4. With some people an aid in the recognition of this position is a contraction of the muscles under the chin.

5. The sound of *x* is usually heard as a combination of *k* and *s* (as in "box" = boks), or of *g* and *z* (as "exact" = egzact), and hence *x* shows a combination of the "undefined" (*un*) and the "tightened narrow" (*tn*) positions; and it is represented thus, *un-tn*.

Summary of Position Eighteenth:
> *The sounds are represented by k, hard g, nk, ng.*
> *The facial appearance is "undefined."*
> *The symbol of representation is un.*

Resolve:

keep = *un-na-ls*	kite	bark	quire	rector
cool		bug	quart	picture
good	caw	wink	cram	location
cow	coy	like	school	whipping
come	camp	talk	scowl	wrapping
curt	get	blank	scrape	fishing
give	game	beg	market	blacking
cute	week	lake	remark	
	look			

Have you the correct answer? = *lo-lt rn-pu tf-el un-st-ep-mo-un-tg lo-tg-tn-el-(ep)?*

I beg your pardon.
Can't you be more careful?
Can't the doctor come today?
We can't see the use of delay.
I can't understand what you say.
What can't be cured must be endured.
Will you take a walk with me?
There's no fun like camping.

I prefer fishing to camping.
I thank you for your trouble.
Did you look under the bureau?
Don't scowl at me in that way.
The early bird catches the worm.
I prefer a film to a plate camera.
I must go to market this morning.
I heard you talking over the scheme.
How did you like the trip to Bermuda?
Where did you have your pictures taken?
The house has a very desirable location.
School opens the first week in September.
They have agreed to arbitrate the strike.
I don't believe in cramming for examination.
Stocks in Wall Street were very irregular today.
I'm glad to hear that the accident was not serious.
What's sauce for the goose is saucy for the gander.
If you will talk more slowly, I can understand you better.

Resolve:

Rufus Choate believed in hard work. When someone said to
him that a certain fine achievement was the result of accident,
he exclaimed, "Nonsense! you might as well drop the Greek
alphabet on the ground and expect to pick up the Iliad."

Resolve:

un-lo-tg	*un-wi-ls-el-tg*
so-na-un	*un-el-tn-tg-el-ls*
tg-ep-lo-un	*un-ag-mo-lt-el-(ep)*
un-lo-+tg-rn	*un-wi-ag-rn-pr*

un-so-tg ls-st-(ep)-tg-rn-un!
un-ep-lo-ls rn-so-ep lo-tg el-+tg ep-el-tg.
un-lo-+tg rn-pu un-el-ls tg-so-ls-wi-ep-st-so?
wi-rn so-rn-pr rn-pu st-ag tn-el-un-tn-mo-tn.
na un-mo-rn-lt rn-tn tg-st-un el so-rn-ls-rn-un.
lo-lt rn-pu mo-lt-el-(ep) ls-rn-tg tg-so un-lo-tg-el-tg-el?
tg-so rn-pu tf-rn-un tf-el ls-lo-tg rn-tn un-ep-mo-rn-tn-rn?

tf-el ls-rn-tn-tg-rn-tn tg-na-tg-tn ls-st-ep un-lo-ls-rn-tg-el-ag.
so-rn-ag rn-pu ls-wi-rn el un-so-st-(ep)-tg el-lt ls-rn-ag-un?
un-ep-rn-tn-ls-el-tn un-el-ls-tn ls-el-tg so-el-tg-tn el + rn-ep.
wi-rn-tg ag-wi-rn-un tg-so ag-rn-lt rn-tg un-lo-ag-rn-lt-st-(ep)-
*   tg-rn-el.*
rn-lt rn-pu + so-tg tn-el-un-tn-na-tg, rn-pu ls-el-tn-tg ls-el-(ep)-
*   tn-rn-tn-tg.*

1. Review the following positions, *na*, *lt*, *ls*, *pu*, *so*, *ᵤi*, *wi-so*, *el*, forming them singly before the mirror, as you do so associating each in your mind with its appropriate sounds.

2. Following is given a drill exercise employing only the positions mentioned in No. 1 above. The positions are given in combinations of one consonant and one vowel position. They are to be read to the pupil first in order, and then repeated promiscuously some six to ten times until mastered. The reader must use either no voice or a voice so low that the pupil may not hear the least whisper. All practice with others must be on this basis, that the pupil cannot hear a sound. (In the following exercises it has not been possible always to give words, and where impossible, manufactured words with phonetic spelling have been resorted to. To make sure, when there might be any doubt about pronunciation, a letter or letters have been given in parentheses, these letters forming with the following or preceding letters a word, and thus showing the sound without question. But in the practice work, the letters in parentheses are not to be sounded.)

fee, fo͞o, foo(t), fah, vow, fuh.
eve, o͞of, oof, ahf, owf, uff.

pea, po͞o, pu(t), pah, pow, puh.
eem, o͞om, oom, ahm, owm, (h)um.

we, wo͞o, woo(l), wah, wow, wuh.

3. Using the mirror, resolve the following:

When the English tongue we speak,
Why is break not rhymed with freak?

Will you tell me why it's true
We say sew but likewise few,
And the maker of a verse
Cannot cap his horse with worse?
Beard sounds not the same as heard?
Cord is different from word;
Cow is cow, but low is low;
Shoe is never rhymed with foe.
Think of hose and dose and lose,
And of goose and yet of choose.
Think of comb and tomb and bomb,
Doll and roll, and home and some.
And since pay is rhymed with say,
Why not paid with said, I pray?
We have blood and food and good.
Mould is not pronounced like could.
Wherefore done and gone and lone?
Is there any reason known?
And, in short, it seems to me
Sounds and letters disagree.

—St. Nicholas

4. Using the mirror, turn the following into English:

*wi-rn-ep-rn-pr ls-so-ag-tn el-(ep) ls-ep-el-lt-el-ep-ls-rn-el-ag.
"tg-mo-lt-el-(ep) ls-rn un-ep-rn-tg-rn-un-el-ag el-lt tf-el ag-mo-rn-
tg-rn-tn," so-el-tn tf-el ls-lo-un-tn-rn-ls el-lt el-tg st-so-ag-tg wi-rn-
pr ls-rn-ep, ep-rn-ls-wi-(ep)-un-el-ls-ag lt-st-(ep) rn-tn wi-ls-rn-pr
tg-so tf-el tn-mo-un-tn. "tf-rn st-so-tg-ag-rn so-mo-rn tf-el-tg
el tg-ep-pu pr-mo-+ tg-ag-ls-el-tg mo-lt-el-(ep) so-rn-ag el-tg-mo-
+ls-tg tg-so ag-so ag-so-un el-tg tf-el lt-st-ag-tg-tn el-lt el ls-ep-rn-
tg-rn +so-ls-el-tg rn-tn tg-so pr-el-tg rn-tn wi-rn-tn."*

—Selected

5. Spend at least one hour in conversation with a friend.
Keep the conversation well in hand yourself so that you will
know the subject.

6. *After* you have resolved the selection under 3 above, have
a friend read it to you.

1. Review the following positions, *ep*, *rn*, *rn-pu*, *wi-rn*, forming them singly before the mirror, as you do so, associating each in your mind with its appropriate sounds.

2. Practice the following exercises, as directed under 2, Lesson 16.

ree, rōō, roo(k), rah, rou(nd), ruh, ri(p), rye.
(p)oor, are, our, ur, ear, ire.

ye, you, you(r), yah, yow, yuh, yea(r).

fi(t), bi(t), wi(t).
if, (h)im.

few, pew.
yoof, yoop.

fie, pie, why.
I've, I'm.

3. Using the mirror, resolve the following into symbols.

Crossed Deaf Tyrant

Paul the First, of Russia, was very deaf, and also very tyrannical. One day an aide de camp, intending to please him, approached and cried into his ear: "I am glad to see, Your Majesty, that your hearing is much improved."

"What is that you say?" growled the Tsar.

Raising his voice, the aide de camp said: "I am glad that your Majesty's hearing is so much improved."

"Ah, that's it, eh?" chuckled the Tsar, and then added: "Say it once more."

The aide de camp repeated the words, thereupon Paul the First thundered: "So you dare to make fun of me, do you? Just wait a while."

Next day the aide de camp was on his way to the mines of Siberia.

4. Using the mirror, turn the following into English.

A Humble Request

"ls-wi, ls-mo-rn wi-rn un-st-so wi-so-tg tg-so ls-ag-mo-rn?"

"tg-st-so; rn-pu ls-el-tn-tg tn-rn-tg tn-tg-rn-ag so-mo-ep rn-pu wi-ep."

ls-st-tn.

"ls-wi, ls-mo-rn wi-rn un-st-so tg-wi-so-tg rn-+tg-so tf-el un-rn-pr-rn-tg?"

"tg-st-so; wi-rn so-wi-+tg rn-pu tg-so tn-rn-tg ls-el-ep-lt-rn-un-tg-ag-rn un-so-wi-rn-rn-tg."

ls-st-tn.

"ls-wi, ls-mo-rn-+tg wi-rn tn-rn-tg el-tg tf-el lt-ag-st-ep el-+tg ls-ag-mo-rn ls-wi-(ep)-ls-ag-tn?"

"wi-rn el-lt tg-st-so-ag-tg rn-pu tg-so-wi-rn-tn tf-el-tg wi-rn· so-wi-+tg rn-pu tg-so tn-rn-tg pr-el-tn-tg so-mo-ep rn-pu wi-ep el-+tg ls-rn un-so-wi-rn-rn-tg, el-+tg wi-rn ls-na-tg rn-un-tn-lo-un-tg-ag-rn so-el-tg wi-rn tn-mo-rn."

ls-st-tn.

"ls-wi, ls-mo-rn wi-rn un-ep-st-so?"

—Selected

5. Spend at least one hour in conversation with a friend.

6. *After* you have resolved the selection under 3 above, have a friend read it to you.

1. Review the following positions, *tf*, *tg*, *ag*, *st*, *st-rn*, forming them singly before the mirror, as you do so associating each in your mind with its appropriate sounds.

2. Practice the following exercises as directed under 2, Lesson 16.

thee, thōō, thah, thou, thuh, thi(ll), thy, thaw, thoy.

eeth, ōōth, ahth, owth, uth, (w)ith, youth, eith, awth, oith.

tea, tōō, too(k), tah, tow(n), tuh, ti(p), tie, daw, toy.

eat, (b)oot, (p)ut, aht, out, utt, it, Ute, ide, awed, oit.

lee, lōō, loo(k), lah, lou(d), luh, li(t), lie, law, loy.
eel, (p)ool, (p)ull, ahl, owl, (h)ull, ill, (m)ule, isle, awl, oil.

faw, paw, waw, raw, yaw.
awf, awp, or.

foy, boy, woy, roy.
oif, oip.

3. Using the mirror, resolve the following into symbols.

Grant stood for the great elementary virtues—for justice, for freedom, for order, for unyielding resolution, for manliness in its broadest and highest sense. His greatness was not so much greatness of intellect as greatness of character, including in the word "character" all the strong, virile virtues. It is character that counts in a nation as in a man. It is a good thing to have a keen, fine intellectual development in a nation, to produce orators, artists, successful businessmen; but it is an infinitely greater thing to have those solid qualities which we group together

under the name of character—sobriety, steadfastness, the sense
of obligation toward one's neighbor and one's God, hard, common sense, and, combined with it, the gift of generous enthusi-
asm toward whatever is right. These are the qualities which
go to make up true national greatness, and these were the
qualities which Grant possessed in an eminent degree.

—Theodore Roosevelt
"The Strenuous Life"

4. Using the mirror, turn the following into English.

*so-el-tg el-lt tf-el ls-mo-tn-tg ep-mo-ls-el-(ep)-tg-na-tn wi-tg
ep-mo-un-el-(ep)-tg rn-tn tf-lo-tg el-lt lt-so-tg (Foote) tf-rn lo-un-
tg-el-(ep). tg-wi-rn-tg-rn-un so-rn-tf tn-el-ls lt-ep-mo-+tg-tn, el
na-tg-rn-tg tg-rn-tn-ls-rn-pu-tg el-ep-st-so-tn ls-rn-tg-so-na-tg rn-
ls-tn-mo-ag-lt el-+tg el rn-el-un tg-st-so-ls-ag-ls-el-tg. tf-el ag-
lo-tg-el-(ep) tn-st-tg tg-so tg-rn-tn-ls-lo-ep-rn-pr lt-so-tg ls-el-rn
lo-tn-un-rn-un rn-ls so-wi-tg rn-tn lt-wi-tf-el-(ep) so-wi-tn.*

"el tg-ep-mo-rn-tg-tn-ls-el-tg," tn-mo-tg lt-so-tg.

*"tf-mo-tg, tn-el-ep, rn-tg-tn el ls-rn-tg-rn na tg-rn-tg tg-wi-tg
ls-mo-rn-un rn-pu so-el-tg."*

*"lo-+tg ls-ep-mo-rn, ag-mo-tg ls-rn lo-tn-un, so-wi-tg so-el-tn
rn-so-ep lt-wi-tf-el-(ep), ls-el-rn ag-st-(ep)-tg?"*

*"ls-wi-rn lt-wi-tf-el-(ep), ls-rn-tn-tg-el-(ep) lt-so-tg, so-el-tn el
pr-mo-+tg-ag-ls-el-tg."*

*"tf-mo-tg, ls-el-rn ag-st-(ep)-tg, rn-tg-tn el ls-rn-tg-rn na
tg-rn-tg tg-wi-tg ls-mo-rn-un rn-pu so-el-tg."*

—Selected

5. Spend at least one hour in conversation with a friend.
6. *After* you have resolved the selection under 3 above, have
a friend read it to you.

LESSON 19

1. Review the following positions, *tn*, *st-so*, *lo*, forming them singly before the mirror, as you do so associating each in your mind with its appropriate sounds.

2. Practice the following exercises as directed under 2, Lesson 16.

see, sŏŏ, soo(k), sah, sou(th), suh, si(t), sigh, saw, soy, so, sa(t).
ease, ooze, (p)uss, ahs, (h)ouse, us, is, use, ice, awes, (v)oice, owes, as

foe, beau, woe, roe, yo(ke), though, toe, lo.
oaf, ope, oath, oat, (h)ole.

fa(t), ba(t), wha(ck), ra(t), ya(m), tha(t), ta(ck), la(d).
aff, am, (c)ar(ry)., ath, at, al(bum).

3. Using the mirror, resolve the following into symbols.

The Gothic church plainly originated in a rude adaptation of the forest trees with all their boughs to a festal or solemn arcade, as the bands about the cleft pillars still indicate the green withes that tied them. No one can walk in a road cut through pine woods without being struck with the architectural appearance of the grove, especially in winter, when the bareness of all other trees shows the low arch of the Saxons. In the woods on a winter afternoon one will see as readily the origin of the stained glass window, with which the Gothic cathedrals are adorned, in the colors of the western sky seen through the bare and crossing branches of the forest. Nor can any lover of nature enter the old piles of Oxford and the English cathedrals without feeling that the forest overpowered the mind of the builder, and that his chisel, his saw, and plane still reproduced its ferns, its spikes of flowers, its locusts, its pine, its oak, its fir, its spruce.

—Ralph Waldo Emerson
"History"

4. Using the mirror, turn the following into English.

el rn-el-un ls-lo-tg lt-ep-el-ls tf-el un-el-+ tg-ep-rn ag-mo-rn-tg-ag-rn lt-wi-ag-el-+ tg-rn-ep-tg rn-tn tn-el-ep-lt-rn-tn-rn-tn tg-so rn-tn-un-st-(ep)-tg el rn-el-un ag-mo-rn-tg-rn st-so-ls lt-ep-el-ls el ls-wi-(ep)-tg-rn. wi-tg rn-tn so-mo-rn na un-el-pr-ag-tg rn-tn ls-ep-mo-rn-tg-tn lt-st-(ep) tn-el-ls rn-+ tg-el-ep-mo-tn-tg-rn-un tg-wi-ls-rn-un el-lt un-wi-tg-lt-el-(ep)-tn-mo-rn-pr-tg, ls-el-tg rn-tg lt-mo-rn-tg; na un-so-tg rn-tg el-ls-el-tg tg-el-tf-rn-un el-+ tg-rn-ag tf-mo-rn ls-mo-tg tn-mo-lt-el-ep-el-ag un-wi-so-tn, so-mo-tg tf-el tn-so-mo-rn-tg tn-mo-tg, so-rn-tf ls-el-pr tn-rn-+ ls-ag-rn-tn-rn-tg-rn el-lt ls-lo-tg-el-(ep): "tg-wi-so, rn-tn-+ tg rn-tg tn-tg-ep-mo-rn-tg-pr, so-el-tg el ls-el-tf-el-(ep)-ag-rn el-ls-rn-ep-el-tg-tn el un-wi-so lo-tn?" tg-so so-rn-pr tf-el ag-mo-rn-tg-rn ep-rn-ls-ag-wi-rn-tg: "wi-rn tg-pu tg-wi-tg tf-rn-un rn-tg tn-tg-ep-mo-rn-tg-pr, tn-el-ep, tf-el-tg el un-wi-so pr-so-tg lo-lt el ls-el-tf-el-(ep)-ag-rn el-ls-rn-ep-el-tg-tn—tg-pu el un-lo-lt."

—After Dinner Stories

5. Spend at least one hour in conversation with a friend.

6. *After* you have resolved the selection under 3 above, have a friend read it to you.

1. Review the following positions, *pr*, *mo*, *mo-rn*, *un*, forming them singly before the mirror, as you do so associating each in your mind with its appropriate sounds.

2. Practice the following exercises, as directed under 2, Lesson 16.

she, shoe, shook(k), shah, chow, shuh, shi(p), shy, shaw, joy, show, sha(d), she(d), shay.

each, oosh, (p)ush, ahsh, ouch, (h)ush, itch, (h)uge, eish, awsh, oish, (c)oach, ash, edge, age.

key, cōō, coo(k), cah, cow, cuh, ki(ck), cue, guy, caw, coy, go, ca(t), ge(t), gay.

eke, (b)ook, ahk, owk, (h)ug, (s)ick, (d)uke, Ike, awk, oik, oak, (h)ag, egg, ache.

fe(d), be(d), we(d), re(d), ye(t), the(n), te(n), le(t), se(t).
eff, epp, air, (B)eth, Ed, ell, ess.

fay, pay, way, ray, yea, they, day, lay, say.
(w)aif, ape, (wr)aith, aid, ail, ace.

3. Using the mirror, resolve the following into symbols.

The scene as the fleet passed out of the harbor must have been singularly beautiful. It was a treacherous interval of real summer. The early sun was lighting the long chain of the Galician mountains, marking with shadows the cleft defiles, and shining softly on the white walls and vineyards of Coruna. The wind was light, and falling towards a calm; the great galleons drifted slowly with the tide on the purple water, the long streamers trailing from the trucks, the red crosses, the emblem of the crusade, showing bright upon the hanging sails. The fruit boats were bringing off the last fresh supplies, and the pinnaces hastening to the ships with the last loiterers on the shore. Out of thirty thousand men who that morning stood upon the decks of the proud Armada, twenty thousand and more were never again to see the hills of Spain. Of the remnant who in two short months crept back ragged and torn, all but a few hundred returned only to die.

—James Anthony Froude
The Defeat of the Spanish Armada,
History of England

4. Using the mirror, turn the following into English.

wi-tg tf-el ls-lo-un-tn el-lt el ep-rn-lt-rn-so-ag-rn-tg tg-rn-ep tn-tg-ep-el-ls-lo-tg (Strabane) rn-tn el tn-tg-st-so-tg so-rn-tf tf-rn-tn tn-rn-un-rn-so-ag-el-(ep) rn-tg-tn-un-ep-rn-ls-pr-tg, rn-+tg-mo-+ tg-rn-tg lt-st-(ep) tf-rn rn-tg-lt-st-(ep)-ls-mo-rn-pr-tg el-lt tn-tg-ep-mo-rn-tg-pr-el-(ep)-tn tg-ep-lo-lt-el-ag-rn-un tf-lo-tg ep-st-so-tg: "tg-mo-rn-un tg-st-so-tg-rn-tn, tf-el-tg so-mo-tg tf-rn-tn tn-tg-st-so-tg rn-tn wi-so-tg el-lt tn-wi-rn-tg rn-tg rn-tn tg-wi-tg tn-mo-rn-lt tg-so lt-st-(ep)-tg tf-el ep-rn-lt-el-(ep)." tf-rn-tn rn-tn tn-el-ls-so-wi-tg tn-rn-ls-rn-ag-el-(ep) tg-so tf-el lt-mo-rn-ls-el-tn lt-rn-un-el-(ep) ls-st-so-tn-tg so-rn-pr so-el-tn rn-ep-mo-un-tg-rn-tg ls-el-rn st-(ep)-tg-el-(ep) el-lt tf-el tn-el-(ep)-lt-mo-rn-el-(ep) el-lt tf-el ep-st-so-tg-tn tn-el-ls +rn-ep-tn el-un-st-so rn-tg un-mo-+tg (Kent): "tf-rn-tn rn-tn el ls-ep-wi-rn-tg-ag ls-lo-tf tg-so lt-mo-rn-lt-el-(ep)-pr-el-ls (Faversham). rn-lt rn-pu un-lo-+tg ep-na-tg tf-rn-tn, rn-pu el-tg ls-mo-tg-el-(ep) un-na-ls tf-el ls-mo-rn-tg ep-st-so-tg."

—*Brooklyn Eagle.*

5. Spend at least one hour in conversation with a friend.

6. *After* you have resolved the selection under 3 above, have a friend read it to you.

1. Have the practice words given in Lesson 1 read to you by a friend.

2. In the following exercises drill is given with a combination of two consonant positions followed by a vowel position. Frequently, however, throughout the exercises, one of the consonant positions will be omitted, as the *ep* position for the *r* sound is frequently omitted in the first of the following exercises, and the *ag* position for the *l* sound is omitted frequently in the second of the exercises. The pupil must watch for this omission of a consonant position. Have each exercise read to you in order, and then repeated promiscuously until the exercise is mastered, that is, about eight to twelve times.

free, fee—froo, foo—frah, fah—Frau, vow—fruh, fuh—fri(ll), fi(ll)—fry, fie—fraw, faw—froy, foy—fro, foe—fra(nk), fa(t)—Fre(d), fe(d)—fray, fay.

flee, fee—flew, foo—flah, fah—flou(t), vow—fluh, fuh—fli(t), fi(t)—fly, fie—flaw, faw—floy, foy—flow, foe—fla(t), fa(t), fle(ck), fe(d)—flay, fay.

bree, be—brew, boo—broo(k), boo(k)—prah, pah—prow, pow—pruh, puh—pri(ck), pi(ck)—pry, pie—braw, pay—broy, boy—bro(ke), beau—bra(t), ba(t)—brea(d), be(d)—pray, pay.

plea, pea—blew, boo—plah, pah—plough, pow—pluh, puh—bli(nk), pi(nk)—ply, pie—plaw, paw—ploy, boy—blow, beau—pla(n), pa(n)—ble(d), be(d)—play, pay.

3. Using the mirror, resolve the following into symbols.

Know you not that our business here is a warfare? And one must watch, and one go out as a spy, and one must fight. All cannot be the same thing, nor would it be better if they were. But you neglect to do the bidding of the Commander, and complain when he hath laid something rougher than common upon you; and you mark not what, so far as in you lies, you are making the army to become; so that if all copy you, none will dig a trench, none will cast up a rampart, none will watch, none will run any risk, but each will appear worthless for warfare.

Again; in a ship, if you go for a sailor, to take up one place and never budge from it, and if you are wanted to go aloft, refuse,—what Captain will have patience with you? Will he not cast you out as some useless thing, and a bad example for the other sailors?

The life of every man is a sort of warfare, a long one and full of divers chances.

And it behooveth a man to play a soldier's part and do all at the nod of his Commander.

—Epictetus

4. Using the mirror, turn the following into English.

el un-el-+ Tg-mo-+ ls-st-ep-mo-ep-rn el-lt ag-st-(ep)-tg tg-rn-tn-ep-mo-rn-el-ag-rn (Disraeli) rn-tg rn-tn ls-na-ls-so-st-ep-tn ep-rn-un-st-(ep)-tg-tn tf-rn-tn rn-+ ls-ep-mo-pr-tg el-lt tf-lo-tg lt-mo-rn-ls-el-tn tg-lo-+ tg-rn-tn ls-el-ep-tn-el-tg-el-ag el-ls-rn-ep-el-tg-tn. rn-pu-pr-pu-el-ag-rn na so-st-ep el tn-ag-mo-rn-tg un-el-ag-el-(ep)-tg lt-mo-ag-lt-rn-tg un-st-so-tg ag-wi-rn-+ tg so-rn-tf tn-lo-tg-rn-tg, ls-el-ep-ls-ag tg-ep-wi-so-tn-el-(ep)-tn so-rn-tf el un-st-so-ag-tg ls-lo-+ tg tg-wi-so-tg tf-rn wi-so-tg-tn-wi-rn-tg tn-na-ls, el tn-un-wi-(ep)-ag-el-tg so-mo-rn-tn-tg-un-st-so-tg, ag-st-un ag-mo-rn-tn ep-el-lt-ag-tn lt-st-ag-rn-un tg-wi-so-tg tg-so tf-el tg-rn-ls-tn el-lt rn-tn lt-rn-un-el-(ep)-tn, so-wi-rn-tg un-ag-el-lt-tn so-rn-tf ls-ep-rn-ag-rn-el-+ tg ep-rn-un-tn wi-so-tg-tn-wi-rn-tg tf-el-ls, el-+ tg ag-st-un ls-ag-lo-un ep-rn-un-ag-rn-tg-tn ep-rn-ls-ag-rn-un tg-wi-so-tg st-so-lt-el-(ep) rn-tn pr-st-so-ag-tg-el-(ep)-tn. so-mo-tg na ep-st-so-tn rn-tg tf-el wi-so-tn, na so-st-ep el ls-wi-tg-ag-un-ep-na-tg lt-ep-wi-un un-st-so-tg, so-rn-tf el so-wi-rn-tg so-mo-rn-tn-tg-un-st-so-tg, un-wi-ag-el-(ep)-ag-rn-tn, lo-+ tg el tg-na-tg-ag-rn-tn tg-rn-tn-ls-ag-mo-rn el-lt un-st-so-ag-tg pr-mo-rn-tg-tn.

—Selected

5. Spend at least one hour in conversation with a friend.

6. After reading the selection under 3 above, but before resolving it, have a friend read it to you.

1. Have the practice words and sentences given in Lesson 2 read to you by a friend.

2. Practice the following exercises as directed under 2, Lesson 21.

three, thee—through, thoo—thrah, thah—throu, thou—thruh, thuh—thri(ll), thi(ll)—thry, thy—thraw, thaw—throy, thoy—throw, though—thra(sh), tha(n), threa(d), the(n) —thray, they.

twee, we—twoo, woo—twah, wah—twow, wow—twuh, wuh— twi(n), wi(n)—twy, why—twaw, waw—twoy, woy— twoe, woe—twa(ng), wha(ck)—twe(lve), we(t)—tway, way.

tree, tea, ree—true, too, rue—trah, tah, rah—trou(t), dou(bt), rou(nd)—truh, tuh, ruh—tri(p), ti(p), ri(p)—try, tie, rye—draw, daw, raw—tro(ve), toe, roe—tra(p), ta(p), ra(p)—trea(d), te(n), re(d)—dray, day, ray.

3. Using the mirror, resolve the following into symbols.

Responsibility alone drives man to toil and brings out his best gifts. For this reason the pensions given to scholars are said to have injured some men of genius. Johnson wrote his immortal Rasselas to raise money to buy his mother's coffin. Hunger and pain drove Lee to the invention of his loom. Left a widow with a family to support, in mid-life, Mrs. Trollope took to authorship and wrote a score of volumes. The most piteous tragedy in English literature is that of Coleridge. Wordsworth called him the most myriad-minded man since Shakespeare, and Lamb thought him "an archangel slightly damaged." The generosity of his friends gave the poet a home and all its comforts without the necessity of toil. Is it possible that ease and lack of responsibility, with opium, helped wreck him? What did the critic mean when he said of a rich young friend, "He needs poverty alone to make him a great painter?" It is responsibility that teaches caution, foresight, prudence, courage, and turns feeblings into giants.

—Newell Dwight Hillis
A Man's Value to Society

4. Using the mirror, turn the following into English.

Seeing the Elephant

ls-rn-tn-tg-el-(ep) ep-el-tg-rn-el-(ep)-tg un-rn-ls-ag-rn-un (Rudyard Kipling) tg-mo-ag-tn el un-so-tg tn-tg-st-ep-rn el-lt rn-ls-tn-mo-ag-lt. so-el-tg tg-mo-rn, na tn-mo-tn, wi-rn so-el-tn tn-rn-tg-rn-un rn-tg ls-el-rn tn-tg-el-tg-rn, rn-tg ag-el-tg+tg (London), so-mo-tg tn-el-+tg-ag-rn el pr-mo-+tg-ag-ls-el-tg el-ls-rn-ep-tg el-tg tf-el tg-st-ep el-tg-el-tg-wi-so-tg-tn-tg, lt-wi-ag-st-so-tg ls-el-rn tg-pu tn-un-pu-ag ls-st-rn-tn. "rn-tn tf-rn-tn ep-el-tg-rn-el-(ep)-tg un-rn-ls-ag-rn-un?" rn-tg-un-so-wi-rn-ep-tg tf-el pr-mo-+tg-ag-ls-el-tg.

"rn-mo-tn," wi-rn lo-tg-tn-el-(ep)-tg.

na tg-el-ep-+tg ep-wi-so-+tg.

"ls-st-rn-tn, tf-rn-tn rn-tn ep-el-tg-rn-el-(ep)-tg un-rn-ls-ag-rn-un."

"lo-+tg rn-tn tf-rn-tn so-mo-ep rn-pu ep-wi-rn-tg?" na un-el-+tg-rn-tg-rn-so-tg.

"rn-mo-tn," wi-rn ep-rn-ls-ag-wi-rn-tg.

ls-st-rn-tn, tf-rn-tn rn-tn so-mo-ep na ep-wi-rn-tg-tn."

lo-+tg ls-rn-lt-st-ep wi-rn el-tg tg-wi-rn-ls tg-so lo-tn-un tf-mo-ls tg-so tg-mo-rn-un el tn-na-tg tf-mo-rn so-el-(ep) un-st-tg, ls-st-rn-tn el-+tg st-ag. wi-rn tn-el-ls-st-so-tn tf-mo-rn lo-tg st-ag ag-rn-tg-el-ep-mo-ep-rn ag-el-tg+tg tg-so tg-pu rn-tg tf-lo-tg so-mo-rn.

—Selected

5. Spend at least one hour in conversation with a friend.

6. After reading the selection under 3 above, but before resolving it, have a friend read it to you.

1. Have the practice words and sentences given in Lesson 3 read to you by a friend.

2. Practice the following exercises as directed under 2, Lesson 21.

spee, pea—spoo, boo—spah, pah—spou(t), pow—spuh, puh—
    spi(t), pi(t)—spew, pew—spy, pie—spaw, paw—spoy,
    boy—spo(ke), beau—spa(t), pa(t), spe(ck), pe(ck)—spay,
    pay.

swee, we—swoo, woo—swah, wah—swow, wow—swuh, wuh—
    swi(m), wi(n)—swi(ne), why—swaw, waw—swoy, woy
    —swoe, woe, swa(m), wha(ck)—swe(ll), we(ll)—sway,
    way.

stee, see, tea—stoo, soo, too—stoo(d), soo(k), too(k), stah, sah,
    tah—stou(t), sou(th), tow(n)—stuh, suh, tuh—sti(ck),
    si(ck), ti(ck)—sty, sigh, tie—staw, saw, daw—stoy, soy,
    toy—stow, so, toe—sta(b), sa(p), ta(p)—ste(p), se(ll),
    te(ll)—stay, say, day.

3. Using the mirror, resolve the following into symbols.

From the Rubaiyat of Omar Khayyam

As under cover of departing day
Slunk hunger-stricken Ramazan away,
    Once more within the Potter's house alone
I stood, surrounded by the Shapes of Clay.

*   *   *   *

Said one among them—"Surely not in vain

My substance of the common earth was ta'en
    And to this figure moulded, to be broke,
Or trampled back to shapeless Earth again."

Then said a Second—"Ne'er a peevish Boy
Would break the Bowl from which he drank in joy;
    And He that with his hand the vessel made
Will surely not in Wrath destroy."

After a momentary silence spake
Some Vessel of more ungainly make:
    "They sneer at me for leaning all awry:
What! did the Hand then of the Potter shake?"

Whereat some one of the loquacious Lot—
I think a Sufi pipkin—waxing hot—
    "All this of Pot and Potter—Tell me then,
Who is the Potter, pray, and who the Pot?"

"Why," said another, "Some there are who tell
Of one who threatens he will to toss to Hell
    The luckless Pots he marr'd in making—Pish!
He's a good Fellow, and 'twill all be well."

4. Using the mirror, turn the following into English.

*lt-ep-mo-+ tg-pr-rn-ls rn-tn tg-so ls-rn lt-lo-ag-rn-so-tg lt-st-
(ep) so-wi-tg tf-rn-ep rn-tn rn-tg rn-tg, tg-wi-tg lt-st-(ep) so-wi-tg
un-el-tg ls-rn un-wi-+ tg (gotten) wi-so-tg el-lt rn-tg. so-mo-tg
tg-pu ls-na-ls-ag el-ls-ep-na-pr-rn-mo-rn-tg na-pr el-tf-el-(ep) ls-
rn-un-st-tn na-pr el-tn lt-wi-so-+ tg tf-rn el-tf-el-(ep) un-el-tg-lt-na-
tg-rn-el-+ tg tg-so lo-lt el-ep-wi-so-+ tg, tf-mo-rn el-(ep) tg-wi-tg
lt-ep-mo-+ tg-tn, tf-mo-rn el-(ep) tn-rn-+ ls-ag-rn el-un-so-mo-rn-
+ tg-el-tg-tn-rn-tn so-rn-tf el ls-rn-tn-tg-rn-tn el-+ tg-el-(ep)-tn-tg-
lo-+ tg-rn-un. tg-so tn-na-un lt-ep-mo-+ tg-pr-rn-ls lt-st-ep rn-tg-
tn rn-so-tg-rn-ag-rn-tg-rn rn-tn el-tn lt-rn-pu-tg-rn-ag lo-tn tg-so
tn-na-un tf-rn mo-+ tg el-lt el ep-mo-rn-tg-ls-st-so lt-st-ep rn-tg-tn
ls-lo-un el-lt un-st-so-ag-tg. el tg-ep-pu lt-ep-mo-+ tg rn-tn st-ag-
so-mo-rn-tn rn-pu-tn-lt-so-ag rn-tg tf-el wi-rn-rn-tn-tg tn-mo-tg-*

tn; ls-el-tg so-na pr-so-tg ls-rn-so-mo-ep el-lt tf-rn-un-rn-un el-lt wi-so-ep lt-ep-mo-+tg-tn lo-tn ls-ep-el-tf-el-(ep) ls-mo-+ls-el-(ep)- tn el-lt el ls-rn-pu-pr-pu-el-ag ls-mo-tg-rn-lt-rn-tg el-tn-st-so-pr- rn-mo-rn-pr-tg, so-rn-tf rn-tg-tn ls-rn-ep-rn-wi-tg-rn-un-el-ag tg- rn-ls-lo-+tg-tn el-+tg tf-ep-mo-tg-tn el-lt tn-el-tn-ls-mo-tg-pr-tg lt-st-(ep) tg-wi-tg-ls-mo-rn-ls-el-+tg el-lt tg-rn-pu-tn.

—H. Clay Trumbull

5. Spend at least one hour in conversation with a friend.

6. After reading the selection under 3 above, but before resolving it, have a friend read it to you.

LESSON 24

1. Have the practice words and sentences given in Lesson 4 read to you by a friend.

2. Practice the following exercises as directed under 2, Lesson 21.

slee, see, lee—sloo, soo, loo—slah, sah, lah—slou(ch), sou(th), lou(d)—sluh, suh, luh—sli(ck), si(ck), li(ck)—sly, sigh, lie—slaw, saw, law—sloy, soy, loy—slow, so, lo—sla(p), sa(p), la(p)—sle(d), se(t), le(t)—slay, say, lay.

skee, see, key—scoo, soo, coo—scah, sah, caw—scow, sou(th), cow—scuh, suh cuh—ski(ll), si(ll), ki(ll)—skew, sue, cue—sky, sigh, guy—scaw, saw, cah—scoy, soy, coy—sco(ld), so, go—sca(t), sa(t), ca(t)—ske(tch), se(t), ge(t)—scay, say, gay.

shree, she—shrew, shoe—shrah, shah—shrou(d), chow—shruh, shuh—shri(nk), chi(nk)—shry, shy—shraw, shaw—shroy, joy—shroe, show—shra(nk), sha(nk)—shre(d), she(d)—shray, shay.

3. Using the mirror, resolve the following into symbols.

A Cuban Teacher's English

The intelligent struggles of the Cuban teachers with English have furnished us with a good many pretty stories. One day not long ago the teachers were invited to some sort of an evening function at the Longfellow House, in Brattle Street. It happened that shortly before the hour for the assembly some ladies who were in front of that house were politely approached by a group of male Cuban teachers, who, with their hats in their hands, stood bowing.

"If you please, dear madams," said their spokesman, "we are invited at this house tonight. We wish to attend. We were been on an excursion to the distance, and have not the time to go to our house. So that we wear, as you see, our day dress. Perhaps you can tell us if it would be permitted to us to go to the reception in our day dress? If it would not, then certainly shall we take the time to go to our house and put on our night dress."

The ladies assured them that they would do much better to go as they were than to put on their night dress, and they bowed gravely and gratefully withdrew.

—Boston Evening Transcript

4. Using the mirror, turn the following into English.

wi-rn ep-na-el-ag-rn ls-rn-ag-na-lt tn-el-ls ls-na-ls-ag tn-mo-rn-lt tf-mo-ep ls-ep-wi-rn-tg tf-st-tg-tn lo-tn ls-na-rn-un tg-pu ls-ep-mo-pr-el-tn lt-st-(ep) un-wi-tg-lt-el-(ep)-tn-mo-rn-pr-tg. so-wi-tg tg-so rn-pu tf-rn-un el-tg el-tg-ls-wi-rn-ep-rn-un lt-ep-mo-+ tg tn-mo-tg tf-rn el-tf-el-(ep) tg-mo-rn tg-so so-el-tg tf-el-tg so-el-tn tg-st-un-rn-un un-so-tg tf-rn-un-tn,—un-so-tg rn-tg-el-lt tg-so ls-ep-rn-+tg? "so-wi-rn," tn-mo-tg na, "rn-pu el-(ep) so-mo-rn-tn-tg-rn-un ls-el-ep-pr-el-+tg-el-ls-ag ag-rn-tg-el-ep-el-pr-so-ep, el un-lo-pr wi-(ep)-tg-rn-un-ag, el-tg tf-el ep-mo-rn-tg, el-tn tg-rn-ep-ag-rn el-tn wi-rn un-el-tg tg-mo-ag, el-lt lt-rn-lt-tg-rn tg-wi-ag-el-(ep)-tn el-tg wi-so-ep." tf-el tg-st-un-el-(ep) tg-so-un rn-ls tg-so tf-el so-rn-+tg-st-so el-+tg lo-tn-un-tg rn-ls tg-so ag-so-un wi-so-tg el-+tg tg-mo-ag so-el-tg na tn-st.

"tg-el-tf-rn-un ls-el-tg el lt-mo-ep-rn tg-el-tn-tg-rn tn-tg-ep-na-tg," na tn-mo-tg, "el-+tg el ls-lo-tg tg-ep-wi-rn-lt-rn-un el tn-ls-ep-rn-un-ag-rn-un ls-el-pr-na-tg tf-ep-pu rn-tg."

"so-wi-rn tg-st-so-+tg rn-pu tg-mo-ag tf-el ls-lo-tg na rn-tn so-mo-rn-tn-tg-rn-un tf-lo-tg so-st-tg-el-(ep)? so-wi-tg +so-tg ls-rn tf-el tn-tg-mo-rn-tg el-lt tf-el wi-rn-so-mo-rn-tn el-lt ag-wi-rn-lt, rn-lt so-na tg-rn-tg tg-wi-tg tg-ep-wi-rn-lt wi-so-ep tf-st-tg-tn-ls-ep-rn-un-ag-el-(ep)-tn tf-ep-pu tf-el-ls so-rn-tf tf-el lt-lo-ag-lt-tn st-so-ls-tg, tn-el-ls-tg-wi-rn-ls-tn?"

—Oliver Wendell Holmes
The Autocrat of the Breakfast Table.

5. Spend at least one hour in conversation with a friend.
6. After reading the selection under 3 above, but before resolving it, have a friend read it to you.

1. Have the practice words and sentences given in Lesson 5 read to you by a friend.

2. Practice the following exercises as directed under 2, Lesson 21.

kwee, we—kwoo, woo,—kwah, wah—kwow, wow—kwuh, wuh —qui(ck), wi(ck)—qui(te), why—kwaw, waw—kwoy, woy—kwoe, woe—qua(ck), wha(ck)—que(ll), we(ll),— kway, way.

Cree, key, ree—crew, coo, rue—croo(k), coo(k), roo(k)—crah, cah, rah—crow(d), cow, rou(nd)—cruh, cuh, ruh— cri(ck), ki(ck), ri(ck)—cry, guy, rye—craw, caw, raw— croy, coy, roy—grow, go, roe—cra(p), ca(p), ra(p)— cre(pt), ge(t), re(d)—gray, gay, ray.

glee, key, lee—cloo, coo, loo—clah, cah, lah—clou(d), cow, lou(d)—cluh, cuh, luh—cli(ck), ki(ck), li(ck)—gli(de), guy, lie—claw, caw, law—cloy, coy, loy—glow, go, lo—cla(p), ca(p), la(p)—gle(n), ge(t), le(t)—clay, gay, lay.

3. Using the mirror, resolve the following into symbols.

American Humor

How a piece of American humor was "managed" is told by the Rev. Dr. Hillis, of Brooklyn. He, with many other American scholars, attended an educational conference at Edinburgh last summer, and sat at dinner beside a Scottish professor.

"I have had some correspondence with Professor B., of Chicago," began the Scotsman. "Is there any possibility of your knowing him?"

"Very well," was the cordial reply, "and he happens to be sitting at the next table, the third man from the end."

"Indeed!" replied the astonished Scot. "I have also had some letters from Professor O., of the University of Michigan. Probably you know nothing of him."

"On the contrary, I know him very well. There he sits, near the corner of the room; the man with whiskers and gold spectacles."

This was too much of a coincidence for the nettled metaphysician, who regarded it merely as American humor; but he went on stiffly:

"Well, sir, I have had relations with another American, a minister near New York, one Dr. Hillis——"

"Oh," laughed back the other, tapping himself on the breast, "I am he."

With a snort of indignation the Scotsman fled the room. As the New York *Tribune* explains, "American humor had been carried too far."

4. Using the mirror, turn the following into English.

tg-so tg-pu wi-so-ep tg-rn-pu-tg-rn—tf-lo-tg rn-tn tf-el tn-el-ls el-+tg tn-el-ls-tn-tg-el-tg-tn el-lt tf-el st-so-ag ls-lo-tg-el-(ep). so-na el-(ep) tg-wi-tg tg-ep-wi-rn-rn-un tg-so tg-pu mo-tg-rn-tf-rn-un rn-tn-ls-mo-pr-el-ag-rn ls-ep-rn-ag-rn-el-+tg st-ep el-tg-rn-pu-pr-pu-el-ag. so-na el-(ep) tn-mo-tg-rn-un wi-so-ep-tn-mo-ag-lt-tn lt-rn-un-st-ep-el-tn-ag-rn el-tg na-pr tg-lo-tn-un el-tn tf-el tg-lo-tn-un el-ep-wi-rn-tn-rn-tn, lo-+tg so-na el-(ep) tg-ep-wi-rn-rn-un tg-so lt-mo-rn-tn na-pr tg-rn-lt-rn-un-el-ag-tg-rn el-tn un-ep-lo-+tg (Grant) lt-mo-rn-tn-tg rn-tg-rn-pu-ls-el-ep-el-ls-ag el-+tg rn-tg-lt-rn-tg-rn-tg-ag-rn un-ep-mo-rn-tg-el-(ep) tg-rn-lt-rn-un-el-ag-tn-rn-tn. tf-el pr-so-ep so-mo-rn tg-so tn-el-un-tn-na-tg. rn-tn tg-so tn-mo-tg el-ls-wi-so-tg wi-so-ep so-el-ep-un rn-tg tf-el tn-ls-rn-ep-rn-tg tf-el-tg ls-wi-(ep)-un-tg tf-lo-tg un-ep-mo-rn-tg tn-st-so-ag-pr-el-(ep): tf-el tn-ls-rn-ep-rn-tg el-lt tg-rn-lt-st-so-pr-tg tg-so tg-rn-pu-tg-rn, el-lt tg-rn-tg-el-ep-ls-rn-tg-mo-rn-pr-tg tg-so tg-na-ag lt-mo-ep-ag-rn, pr-el-tn-tg-ag-rn, el-+tg lt-rn-ep-ag-rn-tn-ag-rn so-rn-tf st-ag ls-mo-tg, lo-+tg el-lt wi-rn-el-(ep)-tg ep-mo-tn-st-ag-pu-pr-tg tg-mo-lt-el-(ep) tg-pu el-ls-lo-tg+tg (abandon) mo-tg-rn tg-lo-tn-un so-el-tg-tn ls-rn-un-el-tg el-+tg-rn-ag rn-tg el-tn

*ls-rn-tg   ls-ep-st-tg   tg-pu   el   tn-el-un-tn-mo-tn-lt-so-ag   el-+tg
tg-ep-wi-rn-el-ls-lt-el-+tg un-el-tg-un-ag-pu-pr-tg.*

—Theodore Roosevelt
The Strenuous Life

5. Spend at least one hour in conversation with a friend.

6. After reading the selection under 3 above, but before resolving it, have a friend read it to you.

1. Have the practice words and sentences given in Lesson 6 read to you by a friend.

2. In the following exercises drill is given with the more difficult vowel positions and those liable to be oftenest confused. These positions, in order of their similarity, are *st* (for the sound of aw), *el-ep* (for the sound of ur), *el* (for the sound of short ŭ, "hut"), *rn* (for the sound of short ĭ, "hit"), *na* (for the sound of long ē, "beet"), *mo* (for the sound of short ĕ, "bet"), *lo* (for the sound of short ă, "bat"), *mo-rn* (for the sound of long ā, "ale"), and *wi-rn* (for the sound of long ī, "isle"). Words have been chosen in which these positions are the only position changed. (Where it has not been possible to find real words, manufactured words with phonetic spelling have been resorted to.) These words have been put in a sentence, the sentence remaining absolutely the same for all the words throughout each exercise except for the one change of position in the chosen word. The pupil should have these sentences read to him, rapidly and naturally, and watch for the change of sound and position. Have each exercise read first in order, and then repeated promiscuously eight to twelve times until mastered. THE WORDS MUST ALWAYS BE GIVEN NATURALLY IN THEIR SENTENCES, AND NEVER ALONE. (Some of the sentences do not make sense, but this is a matter of no importance.)

The awl is sharp.	The fawn is pretty.	The pawn is large.
" earl " "	" fern " "	" burn " "
" (h)ull " "	" fun " "	" bun " "
" ill " "	" fin " "	" pin " "
" eel " "	" feet " "	" bean " "
" ell " "	" fen " "	" pen " "
" Al " "	" fan " "	" pan " "
" ale " "	" fane " "	" pane " "
" isle " "	" vine " "	" pine " "

3. Using the mirror, resolve the following into symbols. (Before doing this, see 6.)

Lawton's Worst Scare

It has been said of General Lawton as of Bayard, that he was never known to be afraid in all his life. Major Putnam Bradlee Strong, who served on the staff of General MacArthur in the Philippines, denies this. He says that General Lawton himself confessed to him that he had been badly scared by bullets, and that very recently.

It happened just beyond the Paco Cemetery in Manila. General Lawton was riding past the cemetery one day with his little boy, when a number of our soldiers were burying some of their comrades. The firing squad found that they had nothing but ball cartridges.

"Oh, they'll do," said the sergeant of the volunteers.

"Ready, fire!" came the order a moment later.

The bullets went whizzing over the grave and over the stone wall, on the other side of which rode General Lawton and his boy, their heads only a few inches below the wall. The bullets made a breeze as they went past.

"That blast of bullets whizzing over our heads scared me blue," said General Lawton, as he related the incident, "but the kid only looked up innocently and asked: 'Say, papa, does it sound like that when you're under fire?' "

4. Using the mirror, turn the following into English.

Went Him Better

rn-tg so-el-tn lo-tg el-tg st-un-pr-tg-ep-pu-ls. tf-el ls-ag-mo-rn-tn so-el-tn un-ep-wi-so-tg-rn-tg, lo-+tg tf-el un-el-ag-mo-un-pr-tg el-lt lt-el-ep-tg-rn-pr-so-ep, wi-(ep)-tg el-+tg ls-ep-rn-un-el-ls-ep-lo-un ls-na-rn-un el-tg-rn-pu-pr-pu-el-ag-rn pr-st-rn-tn tf-el ls-rn-tg-rn-un lo-tg ls-rn-tg lt-mo-ep-rn tn-ls-rn-ep-rn-tg-rn-tg. tg-so-ep-rn-un el-tg rn-+tg-el-(ep)-lt-el-ag el-lt tf-el tn-mo-rn-ag, el ls-lo-tg so-rn-tf el ls-mo-rn-ag el-+tg lo-pr-rn-tg-mo-rn-tg-rn-tg un-wi-so-+tg-rn-tg-el-tg-tn ls-so-pr-tg rn-tn so-mo-rn tg-so tf-rn st-un-pr-

rn-tg-rn-ep-tn tn-wi-rn-tg, el-+tg rn-tg-un-mo-rn-pr-tg rn-ls rn-tg
el so-rn-tn-ls-el-(ep)-tg un-wi-tg-lt-el-(ep)-tn-mo-rn-pr-tg.

ls-ep-mo-tn-rn-+tg-ag-rn na tn-tg-so-tg el-tn-wi-rn-tg, lo-+tg
tf-rn st-un-pr-rn-tg-rn-ep ep-lo-ls-tg el-tg-mo-tg-pr-tg so-rn-tf
rn-tn lo-ls-el-(ep).

"ag-mo-rn-tg-rn-tn el-+tg pr-mo-+tg-ag-ls-rn-tg," na tn-
mo-tg rn-tg el ag-wi-so-tg lt-st-rn-tn, "wi-rn lo-lt tg-pu rn-tg-lt-
st-(ep)-ls rn-pu tf-lo-tg el pr-mo-+tg-ag-ls-el-tg lo-tn ag-st-tn-tg
rn-tn ls-wi-un-rn-tg-ls-so-un un-el-+tg-mo-rn-tg-rn-un lt-wi-rn-lt
el-+tg-ep-el-tg tg-wi-ag-el-(ep)-tn. na st-lt-el-(ep)-tn lt-rn-lt-tg-rn
lt-st-ep rn-tg."

"wi-rn st-lt-el-(ep) so-el-tg el-+tg-ep-el-tg," ep-st-ep-tg el-tg
na-un-el-(ep) lt-st-rn-tn lt-ep-el-ls tf-el ep-rn-ep.

—Selected

5. Spend at least one hour in conversation with a friend.

6. Before even reading the selection under 3 above, have a
friend read it to you.

LESSON 27

1. Have the practice words and sentences given in Lesson 7 read to you by a friend.

2. Practice the following exercises as directed under 2, Lesson 26.

The walk is hard.	He wrought it well.	My yawn is deep.
" work " ".	" rut " "	" yearn " "
" wuck " "	" rid " "	" yun " "
" wick " "	" reed " "	" yeen " "
" week " "	" red " "	" yet " "
" weck " "	" ran " "	" yan " "
" wag " "	" rate " "	" yane " "
" wake " "	" rite " "	
" wyke " "		

3. Using the mirror, resolve the following into symbols. (Before doing this, see 6).

The classic instance of David and Jonathan represents the typical friendship. They met, and at the meeting knew each other to be nearer than kindred. By subtle elective affinity they felt that they belonged to each other. Out of the chaos of the time and the disorder of their lives, there arose for these two souls a new and beautiful world, where there reigned peace, and love, and sweet content. It was the miracle of the death of self. Jonathan forgot his pride, and David his ambition. It was as the smile of God which changed the world for them. One of them it saved from the temptations of a squalid court, and the other from the sourness of an exile's life. Jonathan's princely soul had no room for envy or jealousy. David's frank nature rose to meet the magnanimity of his friend.

In the kingdom of love there was no disparity between the king's son and the shepherd boy. Such a gift as each gave and received is not to be bought or sold. It was the fruit of the innate nobility of both: it softened and tempered a very trying time for both. Jonathan withstood his father's anger to shield his friend: David was patient with Saul for his son's sake. They agreed to be true to each other in their difficult position. Close and tender must have been the bond, which had such fruit in princely generosity and mutual loyalty of soul.

—Hugh Black
"Friendship"

4. Using the mirror, turn the following into English.

An Awkward Name

na so-el-tn tg-ep-mo-tn-tg ag-wi-rn-un el lt-wi-(ep)-ls-el-(ep), lo-+ tg na ag-so-un-tg rn-tg-un-so-wi-rn-ep-rn-un-ag-rn el-tg tf-el un-ag-el-ep-un ls-rn-wi-rn-+ tg tf-el un-wi-so-+ tg-el-(ep) el-lt tf-el pr-na-lt ls-st-so-tn-tg-st-lt-rn-tn, el-+ tg ls-st-rn-+ tg-rn-tg ls-lo-+ tg-st-ls-rn-ls-rn-un-el-ag-rn tg-pu el ls-el-+ tg-ag el-lt ag-mo-tg-el-(ep)-tn tf-el ag-lo-tg-el-(ep) so-el-tn tn-st-(ep)-tg-rn-un st-so-lt-el-(ep).

"so-wi-tg tg-mo-rn-ls?" lo-tn-un-tg tf-el un-ag-el-ep-un.

"ag-wi-so-tg-el-(ep)," tn-mo-tg tf-el lt-wi-(ep)-ls-el-(ep).

tf-el un-ag-el-ep-un ep-rn-ls-na-tg-rn-tg rn-tn un-so-rn-ep-rn rn-tg el tg-st-so-tg un-lo-ag-un-rn-so-ag-mo-rn-tg-rn-tg tg-so tn-tg-wi-(ep)-tg-ag na-lt-tg el-tg-mo-lt ls-lo-tg. ls-el-tg tf-el ls-lo-tg st-so-tg-ag-rn tn-ls-wi-rn-ag-tg el-tg el-tg-ls-na-tg-rn-un tn-ls-wi-rn-ag, el-+ tg tn-mo-tg: "ag-wi-so-tg-el-(ep)."

tf-el un-ag-el-ep-un tg-so-un el ag-st-un ls-ep-mo-tf, el-+ tg tf-el rn-mo-ag tf-el-tg un-mo-rn-ls wi-so-tg so-el-tn ag-wi-so-tg rn-tg-el-lt tg-so so-mo-rn-un tf-el tg-mo-tg.

"tg-st-so el-lt-mo-tg-tn, tn-el-ep, wi-rn st-so-ls? rn-mo-tn, tf-lo-tg-tn ls-el-rn tg-mo-rn-ls—ag-wi-so-tg-el-(ep), tn-el-ep."

"st-so, wi!" tn-mo-tg tf-el un-ag-el-ep-un un-so-wi-rn-tg tn-st-lt-tg-ag-rn. "wi-rn tg-mo-lt-el-(ep) tf-st-tg el-lt tf-lo-tg—rn-mo-tn; rn-ep-tn el ag-mo-tg-el-(ep)."

—*Selected*

5. Spend at least one hour in conversation with a friend.

6. Before even reading the selection under 3 above, have a friend read it to you.

1. Have the practice words and sentences given in Lesson 8 read to you by a friend.

2. Practice the following exercises as directed under 2, Lesson 26.

Your thought is good.			The dawn is here.		
" third " "			" turn " "		
" thud " "			" dun " "		
" thin " "			" din " "		
" theen " "			" deed " "		
" then " "			" den " "		
" yhsn " "			" tan " "		
" thane " "			" Dane " "		
" thine " "			" tide " "		

The lawn is mowed.		
" learn " "		
" lun " "		
" lit " "		
" leed " "		
" let " "		
" lad " "		
" lane " "		
" line " "		

3. Using the mirror, resolve the following into symbols. (Before doing this, see 6.)

I give the story as it was told me, and it was told me for a fact. A man fell from the housetop in the city of Aberdeen, and was brought into the hospital with broken bones. He was asked what was his trade, and replied he was a *tapper*. No one had ever heard of such a thing before; the officials were filled with curiosity; they besought an explanation. It appeared that when a party of slaters were engaged upon a roof, they would now and then be taken with a fancy for the public-house. Now a seamstress, for example, might slip away from her work and no one be the wiser; but if these fellows adjourned, the tapping of the mallets would cease, and thus the neighborhood be advertised of the defection. Hence the career of the tapper. He has to do the tapping and keep up an industrious bustle on the housetop during the absence of the slaters. When he taps for only one or two the thing is child's play, but when he has to represent a whole troop, it is then that he earns his money by the sweat of his brow. Then must he bound from spot to spot, reduplicate, triplicate, sexduplicate his single personality, and swell and hasten his blows, until he produces a perfect illusion for the ear, and you would swear that a crowd of emulous masons were continuing merrily to roof the house. It must be a strange sight from an upper window.

—Robert Louis Stevenson
The Amateur Emigrant

4. Using the mirror, turn the following into English.

A Little Too Soon

el ls-ep-el-lt-mo-tn-el-(ep) so-el-tn un-st-so-rn-un tg-pu rn-un-tn-ls-mo-ep-rn-ls-el-+tg so-rn-tf ag-lo-lt-rn-un-un-lo-tn, so-mo-tg na st-so-lt-el-(ep)-el-ep-tg el tn-tg-rn-pu-tg-rn-+tg tn-mo-rn tf-lo-tg rn-lt na so-el-(ep) tn-rn-ag-mo-un-tg-rn-tg lt-st-ep el tn-el-ls-pr-rn-un-tg na +so-tg tg-mo-rn-un el-tg-lt-lo-+tg-rn-pr el-lt rn-tn tn-el-ls-st-so-tn-tg un-st-so-ls-el tg-so tg-mo-ag tf-el ls-ep-el-lt-mo-tn-el-(ep) so-wi-tg na tf-st-tg el-lt rn-ls.

so-mo-tg tf-el un-ag-lo-tn ls-mo-tg, tf-el ls-ep-el-lt-mo-tn-el-(ep) el-tg-wi-so-tg-tn-tg tf-lo-tg-na +so-tg ag-wi-rn-un, lt-st-(ep) ls-el-ep-ls-el-tn-rn-tn el-lt rn-ag-el-tn-tg-ep-mo-rn-pr-tg, tg-pu el-tg-ls-rn-tg-rn-tn-tg-el-(ep) tf-el un-lo-tn tg-so tn-el-ls ls-mo-+ls-el-(ep) el-lt tf-el un-ag-lo-tn. lt-st-(ep)-tf-so-rn-tf tf-rn-tn tn-tg-rn-pu-tg-rn-+tg lt-wi-ag-el-+tg-rn-ep-tg.

tf-el un-lo-tn ls-el-ag-ls so-el-tn un-el-tg-mo-un-tg-rn-tg so-rn-tf rn-tn ls-wi-so-tf. na ls-ep-rn-tg-mo-+tg-rn-tg tg-so ls-na lt-mo-ep-rn ls-el-pr rn-un-tn-wi-rn-tg-rn-tg, lo-+tg ls-rn-un-lo-tg tg-pu el-ls-rn-pu-tn   tf-el   ls-ep-el-lt-mo-tn-el-(ep)   ep-wi-so-+tg-ag-rn. tf-rn st-so-ag-tg ls-lo-tg ag-mo-tg rn-ls un-st-so wi-tg lt-st-ep el so-wi-rn-ag; ls-el-tg tf-el un-ag-lo-tn ep-st-ep-tg so-mo-tg tf-el ls-ep-el-lt-mo-tn-el-(ep) tn-mo-tg na tg-na-tg tg-wi-tg ls-na tn-st-so rn-ep-rn-tn-ls-wi-tg-tn-rn-ls-ag, tf-el un-lo-tn el-tg tg-wi-tg ls-rn-tg tg-el-ep-+tg wi-tg rn-mo-tg.

—Selected

5. Spend at least one hour in conversation with a friend.

6. Before reading the selection under 3 above, have a friend read it to you.

1. Have the practice words and sentences given in Lesson 9 read to you by a friend.

2. Practice the following exercises as directed under 2, Lesson 26.

I've sawed the wood.			The shawl has gone.		
" surd	"	"	" churl	"	"
" sun	"	"	" shull	"	"
" sit	"	"	" chill	"	"
" seat	"	"	" sheel	"	"
" set	"	"	" shell	"	"
" sat	"	"	" shall	"	"
" sate	"	"	" jail	"	"
" site	"	"	" chile	"	"

I've caught the thief.		
" curt	"	"
" cut	"	"
" keen	"	"
" kid	"	"
" get	"	"
" cat	"	"
" kate	"	"
" kite	"	"

3. Using the mirror, resolve the following into symbols. (Before doing this, see 6.)

It was in the earlier year of my ministry, and my wife and I were invited to dine with one of my good deacons. In that New Hampshire region few laymen were in the habit of asking a blessing at table; but it is quite the custom to invite the minister to do so, and what is customary is looked for. At that time my deafness, though rapidly growing upon me, was in its earlier stages, and I was resolutely striving by special alertness to fight off its natural consequences. So, waiting for the invitation, which surely my reverent deacon would not withhold, I construed a seeming nod to be that, and bowed my head and reverently said grace. Raising my head, I caught the eyes of my wife from across the table, who was looking at me as only wives can look, her face all colors except the right one. It was clearly apparent that something had gone wrong, though I could not divine what. The table was bountifully spread and cheerful, and the hour of conversation after it was very pleasant . . . ; and I quite forgot that reproving glance, that face of many colors. Wives, however, though in many ways useful, can rarely be depended upon to forget; and, reaching home, my ignominy was shown me. The deacon, himself slightly deaf and of soft and muffled voice, was equal to saying grace, even in the presence of his minister, and had done so. That food, like mercy, was twice blessed.

—A. W. Jackson
Deafness and Cheerfulness

4. Using the mirror, turn the following into English.

A Sword Puzzle

tf-mo-rn tf-st-tg ls-st-ep el-lt tf-el ag-na-pr-tg el-lt wi-tg-el-(ep) (Legion of Honor) rn-tg tf-el tg-wi-rn-ls el-lt tf-el lt-el-ep-tn-tg tg-el-ls-st-so-ag-rn-el-tg (Napoleon) tf-el-tg tg-wi-so. tf-rn mo-+ ls-el-ep-el-(ep), rn-tg rn-tn tn-mo-tg, so-el-tg tg-mo-rn ls-mo-tg el-tg st-so-ag-tg so-el-tg-wi-(ep)-ls-tg tn-st-so-ag-pr-el-(ep), el-+ tg lo-tn-un-tg rn-ls so-mo-ep na ag-st-tn-tg rn-tn wi-(ep)-ls. "tn-wi-rn-ep, el-tg st-tn-tg-el-(ep)-ag-rn-tg-tn (Austerlitz)." "el-+ tg so-el-(ep) rn-pu tg-wi-tg tg-mo-un-st-ep-mo-rn-tg-rn-tg?" "tg-st-so, tn-wi-rn-ep." "tf-mo-tg rn-ep rn-tn ls-el-rn un-ep-st-tn lt-st-(ep) rn-pu; wi-rn ls-mo-rn-un rn-pu pr-mo-lt-el-ag-rn-ep." "rn-so-ep ls-lo-pr-rn-tn-tg-rn tg-mo-rn-ls-tn ls-rn pr-mo-lt-el-ag-rn-ep ls-rn-

*un-st-tn wi-rn el-lt ag-st-tn-tg so-el-tg wi-(ep)-ls. so-wi-tg + so-tg
rn-so-ep ls-lo-pr-rn-tn-tg-rn el-lt tg-el-tg rn-lt wi-rn el-tg ag-st-tn-
tg ls-st-so-tf?" "st-so, rn-tg tf-lo-tg un-mo-rn-tn wi-rn pr-so-tg el-lt
ls-mo-rn-tg rn-pu st-lt-rn-tn-el-(ep) el-lt tf-el ag-na-pr-tg." so-mo-
ep-el-ls-wi-tg tf-el tn-st-so-ag-pr-el-(ep) rn-ls-na-tg-rn-el-tg-ag-rn
tg-ep-pu rn-tn tn-st-(ep)-tg, el-+ tg un-el-tg st-lt rn-tn el-tf-el-(ep)
wi-(ep)-ls. tg-wi-so tf-mo-ep rn-tn tg-st-so ls-el-(ep)-tg-rn-un-rn-so-
ag-el-(ep) ep-na-tn-tg tg-so tg-wi-so-tg tf-rn-tn tn-tg-st-ep-rn.
tf-rn st-so-tg-ag-rn un-so-mo-tn-pr-tg rn-tn, wi-so tg-rn-tg na
tg-pu rn-tg?*

—After Dinner Stories

5. Spend at least one hour in conversation with a friend.

6. Before reading the selection under 3 above, have a friend
read it to you.

1. Have the practice words and sentences given in Lesson 10 read to you by a friend.

2. In the immediately preceding exercises drill was given with certain vowel positions. In the following exercises, drill is given with the more difficult consonant positions and those liable to be oftenest confused. These positions, in order of their similarity, are *ag* (for the sound represented by the letter l), *ep* (for the sound represented by the letter r), *tg* (for the sounds represented by the letters, t, d, n), *tn* (for the sounds represented by the letters s and z), *rn* (for the sound represented by the letter *y*), and *un* (for the sounds represented by the letters k, hard g, nk and ng). Words have been chosen in which these positions are the only positions changed. (Where it was not possible to find real words, manufactured words with phonetic spelling have been resorted to.) These words have been put in a sentence, the sentence remaining unchanged throughout each exercise except for the one change of sound and position in the chosen word. The pupil should watch for this change of sound and position. Have the sentences read to you, rapidly and naturally, first in order, and then repeated promiscuously eight to twelve times until mastered. As in the previous exercises, THE WORDS MUST ALWAYS BE GIVEN NATURALLY IN THEIR SENTENCES, AND NEVER ALONE.

A lie	is wrong.	The law	is harsh.	The lap	is soft.
" rye "	"	" raw "	"	" rap "	"
" tie "	"	" daw "	"	" tap "	"
" sigh "	"	" saw "	"	" sap "	"
" guy "	"	" yaw "	"	" yam "	"
		" caw "	"	" cap "	"

3. Using the mirror, resolve the following into symbols.
(Before doing this, see 6.)

How Nye Knew North Carolina

While standing on top of Lookout Mountain a few days ago,
says W. L. Visscher, in the Chicago *Times-Herald*, I was carried
back to the memories of dear old Bill Nye, for we had stood
upon that same spot some years before, and a guide told us that
we could see seven States from that point of view; namely,
Tennessee, Virginia, Kentucky, North Carolina, South Carolina,
Georgia and Alabama.

"Where's North Carolina?" Nye inquired.

The man pointed to a place in the horizon to which distance gave a purple hue.

"What makes you think that is North Carolina?" Nye
asked.

"Oh, we know by the direction and the conformation of the
mountains there," the man replied.

"Well, I know that's not North Carolina," Nye declared,
with some vehemence. "And you know it, too, if you would
stop to think. Here is a map of the United States, and you can see
that North Carolina is pink. Besides, I know it is pink. I live in
that State considerably, and I have helped to paint it red, but of
course I go away sometimes, and it fades a little, leaving it
pin. No sir; you can't stuff me. The place you are pointing at a
color-blind man could see is purple."

Nye said those things so seriously that the man was almost
dazed. He gave Nye a puzzled look, and then went on pointing
out other sister States in the late Confederacy.

4. Using the mirror, turn the following into English.

The Tunnel

un-ep-mo-rn, ep-wi-un tn-tg-ep-pu-tg ls-ag-mo-rn-tg-tn, so-st-ag-
tg rn-tg so-rn-tf rn-pu-ag-rn-tn rn-ag-tn:
el ls-ag-el-ep-tg, tg-so-ls-el-ag-pr-pu-el-tn
un-lo-tg-rn-el-tg: tf-mo-tg tf-el ls-ag-lo-un

pr-st-tn el-lt tf-el tg-el-tg-rn-ag—rn-tg-tn-tg-el-
+ tg tg-wi-rn-tg, tf-el-tg pr-rn-ag-tn
tf-ep-pu tf-el un-ag-st-so-tn-tg so-rn- + tg-st-so-
tn. tg-wi-so-tg tf-rn el-ls-tn-un-rn-so-ep tg-ep-lo-un
ep-el-pr-rn-tn tf-el tg-ep-mo-rn-tg so-rn-tf
ls-ag-wi-rn- + tg, ls-st-tg-wi-tg-el-tg-el-tn
un-ag-lo-ls-el-(ep); tf-el tn-tg-na-ls-tn rn-pu-pr,
rn- + tg-el-(ep)-ls-rn-tg-el- + tg ep-st-ep
un-ep-st-so-tn lt-rn-ep-tn-el-(ep). lo-tn tf-rn-tn
tg-wi-(ep)-un-tg-rn-tn tg-st-so-ag-el-ep-el-tn
tg-st-so mo- + tg?—el- + tg pr-lo-ag so-rn tn-na
tf-el tn-un-wi-rn tg-st-so ls-st-ep?

ls-el-tg ag-so-un! el tn-el- + tg tn-ls-st-so-un-rn
tg-st-tg—el ls-el-ep-tn-tg
el-lt tn-el-tg-pr-wi-rn-tg, el- + tg tf-el lt-wi-(ep),
tn-so-na-tg ls-ag-pu! ls-rn-st-so-ag-tg
el-tg-el-tf-el-(ep) un-el- + tg-ep-rn, lt-mo-ep-el-
(ep) tf-lo-tg tf-el lt-el-ep-tn-tg:
ls-mo-tg-st-so-tn, el- + tg ls-rn-tn-tg-rn + so-tg-
tn el- + tg wi-(ep)-lt-rn-tn-tg-un-st-so-ag-tg,
lo- + tg el tn-ag-st-so ep-rn-lt-el-(ep), lo-tg pu-tn
lt-ag-wi-so-el-(ep)-tg lt-el-ep-pr
tf-el so-mo-tg un-ep-lo-tn lt-ag-el-ep-rn-pr-rn-tn
el- + tg tn-st-so, ls-el-(ep)-lo-ls-tn, so-na ls-mo-rn
el-tg ag-lo-tn-tg rn-ls-el-ep-pr
lt-ep-el-ls tf-lo-tg tg-ep-mo-tg tg-el-tg-rn-ag
so-rn-tf-el-(ep) st-ag ep-st-so-tg-tn tg-mo- + tg.

—William Hurd Hillyer
Lippincott's

5. Spend at least one hour in conversation with a friend.
6. Before reading the selection under 3 above, have a friend
read it to you.

1. Have the practice words and sentences given in Lesson 11 read to you by a friend.

2. Practice the following exercises as directed under No. 2, Lesson 30.

How lame the horse!	The lung is weak.
" rape " "	" rung " "
" tame " "	" tongue " "
" same " "	" sung " "
" game " "	" young " "
	" gung " "

I've lit the light.
" rid " "
" did " "
" sit " "
" kid " "

3. Using the mirror, resolve the following into symbols. (Before doing this, see 6.)

Tissot and the Aloe

Tissot, the distinguished painter, who died recently, while at work on his "Life of Jesus," took extraordinary pains to have every detail absolutely correct, and he flattered himself that he had not made a single error until one day, when he happened to show a critic a water color drawing in which the parable of the barren fig tree was depicted.

Knowing that this drawing was intended to form part of the series entitled "Life of Jesus," the critic examined it very carefully, and finally said:—"I am just wondering why there are so many aloes in this garden. Do you intend the scene to be typical of the time of Christ, or is it an ordinary scene, suitable for any time?"

"My sole object in painting that garden was to depict a familiar scene in the life of Christ," answered the painter, "and I assure you that I have taken the utmost pains not to introduce into the scene anything which would be out of harmony with that epoch."

"Nevertheless, you have made one blunder," replied the critic, "for it is a well-known fact that aloes were not introduced into the Holy Land, nor into any of the countries adjoining the Mediterranean, until after the conquest of Mexico by the Spaniards."

Tissot at once laid aside all other work, and did not rest until he had removed the objectionable aloes from the garden.

4. Using the mirror, turn the following into English.

rn-ep rn-tn el tn-tg-st-ep-rn wi-tg tn-mo-tg-el-tg-el-(ep) tg-rn-ls-rn-pu (Depew) tg-st-so-ag-tg-ls-el-rn pr-st-so-tn-el-lt pr-st-so-tg (Joseph Choate). lo-tg el ep-na-tn-rn-+tg tg-rn-ls-ag-st-ls-lo-tg-rn-un tg-rn-tg-el-(ep) rn-tg ag-el-tg+tg (London), ls-rn-tn-tg-el-(ep) pr-st-so-tg tn-lo-tg tg-mo-un-tn-tg tg-pu el tg-rn-tn-tg-rn-un-so-rn-pr-tg rn-un-ag-rn-pr tg-st-so-ls-ag-ls-el-tg, pu, tg-so-ep-rn-un tf-el un-st-ep-tn el-lt un-wi-tg-lt-el-(ep)-tn-mo-rn-pr-tg rn-tg-un-so-wi-rn-ep-tg:"lo-+tg tg-so so-wi-tg tn-tg-mo-rn-pr-tg rn-tg rn-so-ep un-el-+tg-ep-rn, ls-rn-tn-tg-el-(ep) pr-st-so-tg, tg-el-tn rn-so-ep ls-rn-tn-tg-el-(ep) pr-st-tg-tn-rn tg-rn-ls-rn-pu ls-rn-ag-st-un?"

"tg-so tf-el un-ep-lo-+tg tn-mo-+tg-ep-el-ag tn-tg-mo-rn-pr-tg, ls-el-rn ag-st-(ep)-tg," ep-mo-tg-rn-ag-rn ep-rn-ls-ag-wi-rn-tg tf-el tg-rn-ls-ag-st-ls-lo-tg, so-rn-tf-wi-so-tg el un-so-rn-lt-el-(ep).

tf-rn rn-un-ag-rn-pr-ls-el-tg-tn lt-mo-rn-tn un-ag-wi-so-tg-rn-tg lt-st-ep el ls-st-so-ls-el-+tg so-rn-tf el-tg-tn-el-ep-tg-rn-+tg-rn.

"wi-rn-ls el-lt-ep-mo-rn-tg rn-pu tg-st-so-+tg tg-st-so so-el-tg wi-rn ls-na-tg," lo-tg-rn-tg ls-rn-tn-tg-el-(ep) pr-st-so-tg, el-ls-wi-so-tg tg-so un-st-so tg-so rn-tn ep-mo-tn-un-rn-pu. ls-el-tg rn-tn tg-mo-rn-ls-el(ep) un-so-rn-un-ag-rn tn-ls-wi-rn-ag-tg el un-ag-lo-tg tn-ls-wi-rn-ag el-lt rn-+tg-mo-ag-rn-pr-rn-tg-tn.

"wi! wi-rn tn-na, wi-rn tn-na ls-rn-tn-tg-el-(ep) pr-st-so-tg!"

na rn-un-tn-un-ag-mo-rn-ls-tg. "*ls-rn-tn-tg-el-(ep) tg-rn-ls-rn-pu
ls-rn-ag-st-un-tn tg-so rn-so-ep un-ep-lo-+tg, un-ep-mo-rn-tg
ls-rn-tg-ag un-ag-lo-tn.*"

—*Selected*

5. Spend at least one hour in conversation with a friend, trying to read the lips at about half profile for half of the hour.

6. Before reading the selection under 3 above, have a friend read it to you. After translating the selection under 4 above, have a friend read it to you.

1. Have the practice words and sentences given in Lesson 12 read to you by a friend.

2. Practice the following exercises as directed under 2, Lesson 30.

The leap is long.	They look well.	The loon is wild.
" reap " "	" rook "	" rune " "
" deep " "	" took "	" noon " "
" seam " "	" sook "	" zoon " "
" yeep " "	" cook "	" coon " "
" keep " "		

3. Using the mirror, resolve the following into symbols. (Before doing this, see 6.)

Dogs might well have cherished a warm admiration for Landseer, for no other artist has so skilfully presented their beauty of form and nobility of nature. But as a matter of fact, dogs would have loved Landseer if he had been unable to use pencil and brush, for he loved them, and love begets love.

The great painter respected their rights and resented their wrongs. One of his intimate friends, says the author of "Sir Edwin Landseer, R. A.," wrote that he had a strong feeling against the way some dogs were tied up. He used to say a man would fare better tied up than a dog, because a man can take his coat off, but a dog lives in his forever. He declared that a tied-up dog, without daily exercise, goes mad or dies in three years.

Landseer's wonderful power over dogs is well known. An illustrious lady (whom we may venture to identify as Her Majesty, Queen Victoria) asked him how it was he had gained his knowledge.

"By peeping into their hearts," he replied.

A large party of his friends were with him at his house in St. John's Wood one day. His servant opened the door; three or four dogs bounded in, one a very fierce-looking mastiff.

The ladies recoiled, but there was no occasion for fear. The creature bounded up to Landseer and treated him like an old friend, making the most expansive demonstrations of delight. Someone remarked how fond the dog seemed of him.

"I never saw him before in my life!" said Landseer.

—Youth's Companion

4. Using the mirror, turn the following into English.

so-el-tg na-lt-tg-rn-un rn-tg un-st-so-ag-tg ls-rn-tg-so-rn- + tg-el-(ep), tn-el-ep wi-rn-tn-el-un tg-rn-pu- + tg (Sir Isaac Newton) rn-tg-tn-tg-rn-un-tg-rn-lt-ag-rn tg-ep-pu rn-tn pr-mo-ep lt-mo-ep-rn un-ag-st-so-tn tg-so tf-el un-ep-mo-rn-tg rn-tg so-rn-pr el lt-wi-rn-ep el-tg pr-el-tn-tg ls-rn-tg ag-wi-rn-tg-rn-tg. ls-el-rn tg-rn-un-ep-na-tn tf-el lt-wi-rn-ep ls-rn-un-mo-rn-ls un-el- + ls-ag-na-tg-ag-rn un-rn- + tg-ag-tg, el- + tg tn-el-ep wi-rn-tn-el-un lt-mo-ag-tg tf-el na-tg rn- + tg-wi-ag-el-ep-el-ls-ag el- + tg ep-lo-un rn-tn ls-mo-ag so-rn-tf el-tg-rn-pu-pr-pu-el-ag lt-wi-rn-st-ag-el-tg-tn. pr-wi-tg (John) so-el-tn tg-wi-tg el-tg lo- + tg. el-tg ag-lo-tn-tg na el-ls-rn-ep-tg, ls-el-tg ls-el-rn tf-lo-tg tg-wi-rn-ls tn-el-ep wi-rn-tn-el-un so-el-tn st-ag-ls-st-so-tn-tg ep-st-so-tn-tg-rn-tg.

"ep-rn-ls-pu-lt tf-el un-ep-mo-rn-tg, rn-pu ag-mo-rn-tn-rn ep-lo-tn-un-el-ag!" rn-un-tn-un-ag-mo-rn-ls-tg tn-el-ep wi-rn-tn-el-un, rn-tg el tg-st-so-tg el-lt rn-ep-el-tg-mo-rn-pr-tg lt-mo-ep-rn el-tg-un-wi-ls-el-tg so-rn-tf tf-lo-tg mo-rn-ls-rn-el-ls-ag el- + tg ls-ag-lo-tn-rn-tg lt-rn-ag-wi-tn-el-lt-el-(ep); "ep-rn-ls-pu-lt tf-el un-ep-mo-rn-tg ls-rn-lt-st-ep wi-rn-ls ls-el-ep- + tg tg-so tg-mo-tf!" "ls-ag-na-tn, rn-so-ep wi-tg-el-(ep), ls-wi-rn-tg rn-pu tg-wi-tg ep-lo-tf-el-(ep) tg-ep-st ls-lo-un rn-so-ep pr-mo-ep?" tn-mo-tg pr-wi-tg, el ag-rn-tg-ag so-lo-un-rn-pr-ag-rn. "el-ls-wi-tg ls-wi-rn so-el-ep-tg," tn-mo-tg tn-el-ep wi-rn-tn-el-un, tn-ls-wi-rn-ag-rn-un, "wi-rn tg-mo-lt-el-(ep) tf-st-tg el-lt tf-lo-tg."

—After Dinner Stories

5. Spend at least one hour in conversation with a friend, trying to read the lips at about half profile for half of the hour.

6. Before reading the selection under 3 above, have a friend read it to you. After translating the selection under 4 above, have a friend read it to you.

1. Have the practice words and sentences given in Lesson 13 read to you by a friend.

2. In the immediately preceding exercises the difficult consonant positions were given as initial elements in the words chosen. In the following exercises these difficult consonant positions are given as final elements in the words chosen. In other respects the exercises are similar to the foregoing exercises, and are to be practiced in the same manner.

The pall	is heavy.		Has the "gal"	come yet?
" pour	" "		" " cat	" "
" pawn	" "		" " gas	" "
" pause	" "		" " gag	" "
" balk	" "			

The bell	is loud.
" bear	" "
" pen	" "
" Bess	" "
" peck	" "

3. Using the mirror, resolve the following into symbols. (Before doing this, see 6.)

Bearing a Brother's Burden

Not a few of the returning campaigners at Camp Wikoff were burdened with the weight of two equipments, although they had scarce strength enough to carry one. Why some of them were so heavily laden is indicated by a case related in the New York *Commercial Advertiser*.

A man of the Thirty-third Michigan was loaded down with baggage, and over his shoulder he carried two guns, tied together with twine. He was smoking a cigar, and kept up a constant stream of bantering remarks in a reckless way.

"There's our train, boys," he said, as his company crossed the platform and clambered down the sandy slope toward the siding. "Don't you see the sign? 'Improved Stable Cars.' Well, thank goodness we're going the other way this time."

When the men halted beside the cars, a bystander said affably to this man: "You've got more than your share of baggage."

"I don't know about that," the Michigan soldier answered soberly, all his recklessness vanishing.

"Where did you get the extra gun?"

"It's a dead man's gun. It belonged to a man who was killed down in Cuba."

"And you are taking it home, are you?"

"Yes; I'm taking it to his folks."

The stranger seemed inclined to get more of the story, but the soldier turned his head well away, so that no one could see into his face and read his feelings.

"It belonged to my brother," he said.

4. Using the mirror, turn the following into English.

st-ag-so-mo-rn-tn el-tn ls-el-pr lt-el-ep-pr-pu el-tn tf-rn-ep rn-tn, tn-st-so ls-el-pr el-ls-rn-ep-tn; el-tn ls-el-pr un-so-+ tg-rn-tn el-tn tf-rn-ep rn-tn, tn-st-so ls-el-pr ep-mo-lt-el-ep-el-tg-tn rn-tg un-el-ls-lo-+ tg-tn. st-ag tf-el tg-mo-lt-rn-ag-tn ep-rn-tn-ls-mo-un-tg lt-el-ep-pr-pu. tf-el wi-rn, tf-el pr-mo-tg-el-ep-el-tn, tf-el tn-mo-ag-lt-tg-rn-lt-st-so-tg-rn-tg tn-mo-un-tg so-rn-ag st-ag-so-mo-rn-tn rn-tg-tn-tg-ep-el-un-tg el-+ tg un-el-ls-lo-+ tg ls-lo-tg-un-wi-rn-+ tg. tg-mo-lt-el-(ep) el tn-rn-tg-tn-rn-ep so-el-ep-tg so-el-tn el-tg-el-(ep)-ag-rn ag-st-tn-tg. tg-mo-lt-el-(ep) el ls-lo-un-tg-el-tg-rn-ls-rn-tg-rn lt-mo-ag tg-so tf-el un-ep-wi-so-+ tg. st-ag-so-mo-rn-tn tf-el wi-(ep)-tg el-lt ls-lo-tg un-ep-na-tg-tn el-+ tg el-un-tn-mo-ls-tg-tn rn-tg el-tg-rn-un-tn-ls-mo-un-tg-rn-tg-ag-rn. el ls-lo-tg ls-lo-tn-rn-tn lt-st-(ep) so-wi-tg na rn-tn so-el-ep-tf. so-wi-tg na rn-tn, rn-tg-un-ep-mo-rn-lt-tn rn-tg-tn-mo-ag-lt wi-tg rn-tn lt-mo-rn-tn, wi-tg rn-tn lt-st-(ep)-ls, wt-tg rn-tn lt-st-(ep)-pr-so-tg-tn, rn-tg ag-mo-tg-el-(ep)-tn el-lt ag-wi-rn-tg, so-rn-pr st-ag ls-mo-tg ls-mo-rn ep-na-tg ls-el-tg rn-ls-tn-mo-ag-lt. un-el-tg-tn-na-ag-ls-el-+tg el-lt-mo-rn-ag-tn rn-ls tg-el-tf-rn-un; ls-st-so-tn-tg-rn-un, tg-el-tf-rn-un. tf-mo-ep rn-tn un-el-tg-lt-mo-pr-tg rn-tg tf-el un-ag-lo-tg-tn-rn-tn el-lt wi-so-ep wi-rn-tn, rn-tg wi-so-ep tn-ls-wi-rn-ag-tn, rn-tg tn-lo-ag-rn-so-tg-mo-rn-pr-tg-tn, el-+tg tf-el un-ep-lo-tn-ls el-lt lo-+tg-tn. rn-tn tn-rn-tg ls-rn-tg-st-ls-tn rn-ls, ls-wi-(ep)-tn st-ag rn-tn un-so-tg rn-+ls-ep-mo-pr-tn. ls-mo-tg tg-st-so tg-wi-tg so-wi-rn tf-mo-rn tg-so tg-wi-tg tg-ep-el-tn-tg rn-ls; ls-el-tg tf-mo-rn tg-so tg-wi-tg tg-ep-el-tn-tg rn-ls. rn-tn lt-wi rn-tn un-ag-lo-tn-rn-tn rn-tn wi-rn, tg-rn-ls-na-tg-tn rn-tn pr-na-un, ls-rn-tg-pr-rn-tn tf-el tg-st-so-tn, tn-mo-tg-tn tf-el ls-wi-(ep)-un el-lt tf-el ls-na-tn-tg wi-tg tf-el ls-lo-un el-lt tf-el mo-tg, el-+tg ep-wi-rn-tg-tn, st-so lt-pu-ag! st-so lt-pu-ag! wi-tg tf-el lt-wi-ep-el-tg el-lt el un-rn-un.

—Ralph Waldo Emerson
Spiritual Laws

5. Spend at least one hour in conversation with a friend, trying to read the lips at about half profile for half of the hour.

6. Before reading the selection under 3 above, have a friend read it to you. After translating the selection under 4 above, have a friend read it to you.

1. Have the practice words and sentences and the anecdotes given in Lesson 14 read to you by a friend.

2. Practice the following exercises as directed under 2, Lesson 33.

The mull	is warm.		The pill	is small.		The meal	is ready.
" myrrh	"	"	" pier	"	"	" beet	"	"
" mud	"	"	" pit	"	"	" peace	"	"
" muss	"	"	" miss	"	"	" peak	"	"
" mug	"	"	" pick	"	"		

3. Using the mirror, resolve the following into symbols. (Before doing this, see 6.)

The American Soldier

The American soldier in the ranks has brains. It used to be thought that a soldier's only duty was to obey specific orders to the letter. The American soldier is supposed to think. The result is that where three orders would be necessary to obtain a certain result with a platoon of Russian peasants, the American soldier requires but one, and infers the other two.

The permission and the necessity to think is American through and through, and finds expression fitly enough in Mr. Carnegie's advice to "break rules for the good of the firm." When an American is advancing in open order or on the skirmish-line, he is often trusted to fight his own fight in his own way. He is expected to use his head.

One regiment in Luzon was able to take entire charge of the repairing and running of the Manila and Dagupan railroad. In the ranks were experienced civil and mechanical en-

gineers, train crews, linemen, telegraph operators, train des-
patchers, switchmen—indeed, all the men necessary to a railroad system.

The start of one of these trains was an example of the
American's free and easy humor. The engine-driver in blue jean
overalls and leather cap, would lean from the window of the
"dummy" cab; the fireman would look back with the bell
rope in his hand, and some wit of the ranks, who played con-
ductor, with two hundred rounds swung from his belt and a
revolver instead of a ticket punch, would wave his arms and cry:

"All aboard for the Northern Limited, stopping at Malolos
and Calumpit, junction of the railroad and the dirt road."

—*McClure's* magazine

4. Using the mirror, turn the following into English.

*tg-rn-ls-wi-un-ep-el-tn-rn el-tn tg-wi-tg st-so-tg-ag-rn tg-st-tg
tf-rn el-ls-mo-ep-rn-un-el-tg-tn wi-so tg-so rn-pu-tn ag-rn-ls-el-(ep)
-tg-rn so-rn-tf-wi-so-tg el-ls-rn-pu-tn-rn-un rn-tg, el-+ tg wi-so
tg-so tn-rn-un-rn-so-ep rn-un-so-wi-ag-rn-tg-rn: rn-tg el-tn st-ag-
tn-st-so tg-st-tg tf-el-ls lt-ep-el-tg-el-ep-tg-rn-tg-rn. tf-lo-tg so-el-
ep-tg el-tn un-st-tg wi-so-tg el-lt lt-lo-pr-tg rn-tg tf-rn st-so-ag-tg
so-el-ep-ag-tg, el-+ tg tg-st-so so-el-+ tg-el-(ep), un-el-tg-tn-rn-tg-
el-ep-rn-un so-el-tg so-el-tn tg-el-tg rn-tg rn-tg-tn tg-mo-rn-ls rn-tg
1793, un-el-tg-tn-rn-tg-el-ep-rn-un st-ag-tn-st-so tf-el-tg rn-tg tn-
tg-rn-ag lt-rn-un-rn-so-ep-tn rn-tg tf-el ls-ep-st-so-un-ep-lo-ls el-lt
el-tn-lo-tn-rn-tg-tn. tg-mo-lt-el-(ep)-tf-el-ag-mo-tn tf-mo-ep rn-tn
rn-tg tf-el rn-so-tg-wi-rn-tg-rn-tg tn-tg-mo-rn-tg-tn el tn-st-(ep)-tg
el-lt un-wi-rn-+ tg-ag-rn-tg-rn-tn, el tn-mo-tg-tn el-lt rn-pu-ls-
el-tg lt-mo-ag-st-so-pr-rn-ls, el ep-mo-un-el-un-tg-rn-pr-tg el-lt
tf-el tg-rn-pu-tg-rn el-lt ls-rn-pu-pr-pu-el-ag mo-ag-ls st-so-tg ls-el-
rn ls-lo-tg tg-so ls-lo-tg, tn-tg-ep-st-un-el-(ep) tf-el-tg mo-tg-rn-so-
mo-ep rn-tg tf-rn st-so-ag-tg so-el-ep-ag-tg, el-+ tg tn-el-ep-tg-rn-
tg-ag-rn tn-tg-ep-st-un-el-(ep) tf-el-tg rn-tg tf-rn el-ls-el-(ep) st-(ep)
ls-rn-tg-ag un-ag-lo-tn-rn-tn el-lt rn-un-ag-el-+ tg, lt-ep-lo-tg-tn,
st-(ep) pr-el-ep-ls-el-tg-rn. tf-el tg-lo-pr-so-ep-el-ag rn-+ ls-el-ag-tn
el-lt mo-lt-ep-rn tn-rn-tg-rn-tn-tg rn-tg el-ls-mo-ep-rn-un-el rn-tn
tg-so ep-rn-tn-ls-mo-un-tg mo-lt-ep-rn el-tf-el-(ep) tn-rn-tg-rn-tn-
tg, lo-+ tg tg-so lt-na-ag tf-el-tg tn-rn-tg-rn-tn-tg-pr-rn-ls un-wi-*

tg-tn-tg-rn-tg-rn-pu-tg-tn el tn-el-ep-tg-rn-tg un-ep-wi-so- + tg el-lt ep-rn-tn-ls-mo-un-tg. tf-rn wi-rn-tg-na-el el-lt na-pr ls-lo-tg-tn na-un-so-el-ag ep-wi-rn-tg-tn rn-tn tn-st-so lt-so-ag-rn ep-na-el-ag-wi-rn-tn-tg tf-el-tg tf-el ep-rn-pr st-(ep) ls-wi-so-el-(ep)-lt-so-ag ls-lo-tg lt-na-ag-tn rn-tg tg-st-so rn- + tg-rn-un-tg-rn-tg-rn tg-so tg-mo-rn-un rn-tn tg-el-ep-tg el-ls-el-un tf-el un-ep-wi-so-tg, el- + tg tg-el-tn tg-wi-tg rn-un-tn-ls-mo-un-tg mo-tg-rn tg-mo-lt-el-ep-el-tg-tn lt-ep-el-ls tf-el ls-so-ep-rn-tn-tg.

—James Bryce
The American Commonwealth

5. Spend at least one hour in conversation with a friend, trying to read the lips at about half profile for a quarter of the hour, and at full profile for another quarter of the hour.

6. Before reading the selection under 3 above, have a friend read it to you. After translating the selection under 4 above, have a friend read it to you.

LESSON 35

1. Have the practice words and sentences and the anecdote given in Lesson 15 read to you by a friend.

2. Practice the following exercises as directed under 2, Lesson 33.

His pull	is strong.		The tool	is sharp.	
" poor	"	"	" toot	"	"
" put	"	"	" tōōs	"	"
" puss	"	"	" dōōk	"	"
" book	"	"			

3. Using the mirror, resolve the following into symbols. (Before doing this, see 6.)

. . . Was this grass of the earth made green for your shroud only, not for your bed? And can you never lie down *upon* it, but only *under* it? The heathen, in their saddest hours, thought not so. They knew that life brought its contest, but they expected from it also the crown of all contest: No proud one! no jewelled circlet flaming through Heaven above the heights of the unmerited throne; only some few leaves of wild olive, cool to the tired brow, through a few years of peace. It should have been of gold, they thought; but Jupiter was poor; this was the best the god could give them. Seeking a better than this, they had known it a mockery. Not in war, not in wealth, not in tyranny, was there any happiness to be found for them—only in kindly peace, fruitful and free. The wreath was to be of *wild* olive, mark you:- the tree that grows carelessly, tufting the rocks with no vivid bloom, no verdure of branch; only with soft snow of blossoms, and scarcely fulfilled fruit, mixed with gray leaf and thornful stem; no fastening of diadem for you but with such sharp embroidery. But this, such as it is, you may win, while yet you

live; type of gray honor and sweet rest. Free-heartedness, and
graciousness, and undisturbed trust, and requited love, and the
sight of the peace of others, and the ministry to their pain; these,
—and the blue sky above you, and the sweet waters and flowers
of the earth beneath; and mysteries and presences, innumerable,
of living things,—may yet be here your riches; untormenting
and divine: serviceable for the life that now is; nor, it may be,
without promise of that which is to come.

—John Ruskin
The Crown of Wild Olive

4. Using the mirror, turn the following into English.

*so-na el-ep st-ag ep-mo-tg-rn tg-so ag-lo-lt el-tg tf-el ls-ag-wi-
so-ls-el-tg el-ls-el-un ag-st-(ep)-tg-tn; so-na pr-so-tg un-el-tg-tn-rn-
tg-el-(ep) st-ag-tn-st-so tf-el un-mo-rn-tn el-lt el ag-st-(ep)-tg
el-ls-el-un tf-el ls-ag-wi-so-ls-rn-tg. wi-rn-lt tn-na-tg el ag-st-rn-el-
(ep) rn-tg tf-el wi-so-tn el-lt el mo-ls-ep-rn-tg-na-el-tg lt-rn-pr-el-
(ep)-ls-el-tg; el-+tg wi-rn tg-st-so, ls-el-tg tg-el-tf-rn-un so-rn-ag
rn-+tg-rn-pu-tn ls-na tg-so tg-rn-tn-un-ag-st-so-tn, so-rn-pr el-lt
tf-na-tn tg-pu so-el-tn tf-el ls-mo-tg-el-(ep) pr-mo-+tg-ag-ls-el-tg.
tn-el-ls el-lt wi-so-ep lt-wi-rn-tg-rn-tn-tg ls-rn-mo-rn-lt-rn-el-(ep),
tf-st-so rn-tg ag-so-un-tn so-mo-ag rn-tg-el-lt lt-ep-el-ls tf-el ls-wi-
un-tn-rn-tn, ls-mo-rn tn-na-ls na-lt-tg ls-ep-pu-tg-el-ag tg-so tf-el
un-lo-ag-el-ep-rn. so-na ls-st-so-tn-tg tg-pu st-lt-tg ls-lo-tg-el-(ep)-
tn tf-el-tg el-(ep) ls-el-ep-st-so-un-rn-el-ag ep-lo-tf-el-(ep) tf-el-tg
rn-pu-tg-rn-lt-el-ep-tn-el-ag; tf-lo-tg, ag-wi-rn-un el un-el-+tg-ep-
rn so-wi-rn-tg, so-rn-ag tg-wi-tg ls-mo-ep tg-ep-lo-tg-tn-ls-st-(ep)-
tg-mo-rn-pr-tg lt-st-ep el el-+tg-ep-el-tg ls-wi-rn-ag-tn, tg-st-(ep)
lt-ep-el-ls tf-el ls-wi-(ep)-ag-el-(ep) tg-so tf-el un-rn-pr-rn-tg. tg-
so ls-na el pr-mo-+tg-ag-ls-el-tg rn-tn tg-so ls-na so-el-tg st-ag
tf-el so-el-ep-ag-tg st-so-lt-el-(ep), el-+tg rn-tg mo-lt-ep-rn ep-rn-
ag-mo-rn-pr-tg el-+tg un-ep-mo-rn-tg el-lt tn-st-tn-wi-rn-rn-tg-rn.
rn-tg rn-tn el wi-rn un-st-ag-rn-un, tg-so so-rn-pr el ls-lo-tg
ls-el-tn-tg lt-el-ep-tn-tg ls-rn ls-st-(ep)-tg, el-+tg tf-mo-tg tg-rn-lt-
st-so-tg rn-ls-tn-mo-ag-lt lt-st-(ep) ag-wi-rn-lt. lo-+tg,el-tg-lo-ls-
rn-ag-rn, tf-el ls-lo-tg-el-(ep)-tn el-lt el tn-el-ep-tg-rn-tg tn-st-so-un-
st-ag-tg el-ls-el-(ep) un-ep-mo-rn-tg lo-lt el un-wi-rn-+tg el-lt
un-el-ep-el-tg-tn-rn, el-+tg ls-na-tg so-rn-tf el tn-el-ep-tg-rn-tg*

rn-un-tn-tg-el-ep-tg-el-ag lo-un-tn-mo-ls-tg-mo-rn-pr-tg tf-ep-pu-
wi-so-tg st-ag tf-rn el-tf-el-(ep)-tn, el-+tg tf-rn-tn tg-mo-+tg-tn
tg-so un-na-ls el-tn so-mo-ag tn-lo-tg-rn-tn-lt-wi-rn-tg so-rn-tf
tn-ag-wi-rn-tg el-un-so-wi-rn-ep-ls-el-+tg-tn. . . . ls-el-tg ls-lo-tg-
el-(ep)-tn, ag-wi-rn-un wi-(ep)-tg, pr-so-tg ls-rn rn-pu-ls-el-tg el-+
tg tn-mo-+tg-ep-el-ag.

—Robert Louis Stevenson
The Amateur Emigrant

5. Spend at least one hour in conversation with a friend, trying to read the lips at about half profile for a quarter of the hour,
and at full profile for another quarter of the hour.

6. Before reading the selection under 3 above, have a friend
read it to you. After translating the selection under 4 above,
have a friend read it to you.